GODDESSES ARE AGELESS

The Girlfriends' Guide to Health, Happiness, and Vitality at Any Age

Yvonne Aileen

800 Muses Publishing

To Goddess Kathy, my sister.
May this book inspire you to live your life boldly.
And to my sister Goddesses everywhere.
May it do the same for you.

publisher@800Muses.com
www.800Muses.com

Ordering Information:

Quantity sales. Special discounts are available on quantity purchases by corporations, associations, and others. For details, contact the "Special Sales Department" at the address above.

Goddesses Are Ageless: The Girlfriends' Guide to Health, Happiness, and Vitality at Any Age / Yvonne Aileen. —1st ed.

ISBN: 978-1-7369105-4-2

GODDESSES ARE AGELESS

WELCOME, GODDESS

You can be gorgeous at thirty, charming at forty, and irresistible for the rest of your life. ~ Coco Chanel

A friend recently posted on Facebook that at age 55, she was proud of where she was in her life:

> I find myself, for the first time, making plans for MY future. I have all the experience and knowledge from years of digging and travelling the underground, I now can take the time to muse, to choose, to start through a door of my own creativity. I am alive, I am a creator, I have talent, now, what will I be?

This is how we should all face our better half, the second half of life. We can enjoy a new softening, a new patience, a new calm, a new wisdom. We can take our nose off the grindstone and PLAY. And you've earned it, Goddess.

Facing Aging

Bette Davis said, "Old age ain't no place for sissies."

A few minutes after arriving at my 20-year high school reunion, having found no one I recognized, I approached two men standing together and said, "This is embarrassing. I don't recognize anyone." In chorus, they said, "Yvonne!" It turned out they were members of a future business leaders group I had been involved with. I felt bad that I'd not recognized them, but I was surprised how much they had changed in 20 years.

Ten years later, at my 30-year high school reunion, I texted a friend who was on her way to confirm I was in the right place. My first thought had been that I'd come to a reunion for my parents. Thirty years can take its toll. And so can 40.

I recently showed a dear friend a photo of a woman who I felt looked 20 years older than me and told my friend that she and I were the same age, expecting her to be shocked. But my friend said, "So?"

Ouch.

Is it possible we have prosopagnosia (facial blindness) for our own faces, seeing them as we *were* rather than as we *are*? Profiles on dating apps frequently read, "People say I look younger than my age." But how often is this true? I don't *feel* my age—60 at the time of this writing—and although I feel like I don't look it, I probably do. Besides, what is 60 supposed to look like?

Melanie Griffith famously said we shouldn't lie about our age, we should defy it. But why do either? Women over 50 (or 60 or 100) aren't clones. Why then are we bombarded with "hairstyles for women over 50" and "fashion for women over 50"? Let's celebrate our individuality *and* every single candle on our birthday cakes. At the time of this writing, Emma Thompson is 62, Christie Brinkley is 68, Meryl Streep is 72, Cher is 75, Helen Mirren is 76, Tina Turner is 82, and Judy Dench is 87. Each lives life on her own terms. Betty White was 99 when she passed and was still a bawdy, vivacious, active, and widely adored woman. We all have the ability to rock our lives, regardless of age.

The Birth of the Book

This book contains everything I've learned and know about living life full-out, healthy, and fulfilled. For more than two decades, I've been immersing myself in longevity research. My goal is to stay healthy into the triple digits. My youngest son was diagnosed with autism at age two and a half, and being his mom is both a privilege and a responsibility. He is kind and creative and gentle, and knowing there will be a time when I won't be there for him terrifies me. While we work on his independence and life skills, I work on maximizing my health span. There is so much we can do to live with vibrancy and good health.

Also fueling my desire for a longer health span are the people I love who are dealing with (or lost their battle with) illness and disease. Their conditions remind me how lucky I am to have my health. When I think about skipping a workout, I remember that not everyone *can* work out. And when I think about eating crap, I remember that putting poison in my body is taking my health for granted and I have no right to do that. I slip up, sure. But I always get back on track.

And what's the point of living longer if you're unhappy? *Goddesses Are Ageless* is also about living the life we're meant to live. This involves honoring our goals and dreams and taking charge of our mental health, our relationships, and our attitude toward life. We are all connected and the fact you're reading this book means you're also looking for a way to live your best life. I celebrate you for that! Although we are each born into different life circumstances and into family dynamics we had little control over, by the time we reach midlife, we receive a beautiful gift every single day: We get to choose how we want to live the rest of our lives.

CHAPTER ONE

THE AGELESS GODDESS

ROCKING THE SECOND HALF

Do not grow old, no matter how long you live. Never cease to stand like curious children before the great mystery into which we were born. ~ Albert Einstein

How old are you? If you answer with your *chronological* age, that's one truth. But you also have a *biological* age, determined by the state of your organs, immune system, heart, chromosomes, and other markers, and this may be older or younger than your chronological age. In a New Zealand study, researchers found that the biological age of 38-year-old participants ranged from 30 to 60! (1)

While our chronological age ratchets up relentlessly year after year, we have remarkable control over our biological age. This is the secret to living healthier longer. Aging occurs at the cellular and hormonal levels. Let's look at how we can slow, and even reverse, these biological aging processes.

Cellular Aging

When cells are damaged by oxidative stress (caused by free radicals) they turn over, or replicate. (This is called cell division.) They can only do this about 50 or 60 times before replication fails and the cell dies. Genes within cells are protectively encased in chromosomes, which tightly wrap around them. **Telomeres** are structures at the ends of chromosomes that act like the plastic caps on shoelaces. But each time a cell divides, its telomere shortens. When telomeres become short enough that the genes they protect could be damaged, the cell stops dividing and renewing. This causes cellular aging. Both genetics and lifestyle choices can contribute to telomere shortening. So can stress.

Chronic inflammation also plays a role in cellular death. **Inflammaging** is the term for chronic, low-grade inflammation because of its relationship to biological aging. While inflammation is necessary for healing—helping the body fight injury and infection—chronic inflammation is destructive. The immune system cells that normally protect us go into overdrive and may begin to destroy healthy cells in arteries, organs, and joints. Early signs of inflammaging are hard to spot because they're subtle at first (fatigue is a common early signal). Eventually, though, inflammaging can lead to heart disease, vascular disease, diabetes, obesity, cancer, Alzheimer's, arthritis, and other age-related diseases.

"Inflammaging is a highly significant risk factor for both morbidity and mortality in the elderly people, as most if not all age-related diseases share an inflammatory pathogenesis." ~ *The Journal of Gerontolology, June 2014 (2)*

Hormonal Aging

Hormones are chemical substances that act as messengers and crew bosses, controlling and coordinating activities throughout the body, such as helping to build bones and muscle. They can also contribute to emotional and mental health. Sedentary lifestyles and the Standard American Diet (SAD) can negatively affect the hormonal environment. When hormone output decreases, this can lead to changes in the skin (wrinkles, loss of elasticity), loss of muscle tone, decreased bone density, and changes to our sex organs and drive. For instance, as women approach menopause, a decrease in estrogen leads to a decrease in vaginal fluids, and sexual tissues begin to atrophy. As men age, their testosterone levels decrease, leading to a decrease in lean muscle and sperm production.

Age-Related Disease

"I don't want to live to be 100," some say. The reason is that they associate a longer lifespan with cognitive decline and frailty. But these are not inevitable. Consider the following forms of age-related disease for which lifestyle is a significant determining factor:

- **Cardiovascular disease**, especially coronary artery disease, which involves a narrowing or blockage of the arteries that supply blood to the heart.
- **Stroke (cerebrovascular disease)** caused when blood stops flowing in one area of the brain because of a disruption of one of the blood vessels. This deprives brain cells of oxygen, and they begin to die very quickly. Strokes may be either ischemic (any lack of blood flow to the brain) or hemorrhagic (caused by a rupture of a blood vessel, resulting in bleeding in the brain).
- **High blood pressure (hypertension),** measured by the amount of force blood exerts on the walls of your arteries when your heart pumps.
- **Cancer,** the runaway growth of abnormal cells.
- **Type 2 diabetes**, a disorder in how your body uses glucose from food and involves insulin resistance.
- **Parkinson's disease**, a progressive neurological disorder involving tremors, stiffness, and halting movement. (It's believed that genetics and environmental factors are causal here, including exposure to toxins. Traumatic brain injuries, such as from an automobile accident, can also be a cause.)

- **Dementia,** including Alzheimer's disease, which causes a loss of brain function and may involve memory loss, mood changes, confusion, difficulty communicating, and poor judgment.
- **Chronic obstructive pulmonary disease (COPD),** a reduction of airflow into and out of the lungs due to inflammation in the airways, thickening of the lining of the lungs, and an over-production of mucus in the air tubes. Lifestyle causes include smoking (including second-hand smoke), occupational contaminants, and industrial pollution.
- **Osteoarthritis**, a degenerative joint disease, and the most common form of arthritis. Risk factors include genetics, obesity, and prior joint injury.
- **Osteoporosis**, known as "brittle bone disease," and characterized by loss of bone mass, leading to thinner, weaker bones. Vitamin D deficiency is common in those afflicted. Ways to prevent it include a diet rich in calcium and vitamin D, not smoking, and doing regular weight-bearing exercise.
- **Cataracts**, a progressive cloudiness in the lens of the eye that may be associated with exposure to UV light, smoking, and diabetes. Surgical correction, if necessary, is straightforward and involves removing and replacing the lens.
- **Age-related macular degeneration**, which makes it difficult to see objects directly in front of you, although peripheral vision is often unaffected. Risk factors besides age include smoking, race (Caucasians are more susceptible) and family history.
- **Hearing loss**, which occurs due to the deterioration of tiny hairs within your ears that help process sound. Almost 50% of those over age 75 have disabling age-related hearing loss.

The Good News

Aging itself is not a disease, merely a risk factor for age-related diseases, and these are not preordained. Inflammation, environmental exposure to pollutants and radiation, and lifestyle factors such as smoking, a poor diet, stress, and a lack of exercise are also contributing factors. You have control over nearly all of these—you can also take steps to **reverse** your current biological age with lifestyle changes. And while nearly all adults over age 65 have at least one chronic disease, and 50% have at least two, you can lower your risk of developing the most common age-related diseases by as much as 80% with simple lifestyle choices. This is the power of Goddess living. Let's look now at how we can reverse cellular, hormonal, and metabolic aging.

Reversing Cellular Aging

By minimizing the number of times cells must replicate, we can slow down the effects of cellular aging. The right lifestyle choices (eating healthy, reducing toxins, getting appropriate fresh air and exercise, and stress reduction) can lengthen telomeres. Studies have found that it can take as little as one to six months of mental or physical training to elongate telomeres. NASA did a study with twins that showed telomeres lengthening in space, shortening on a return to Earth, and then normalizing after six months, proving that lengthening telomeres is possible. (3) Lengthening telomeres is biological reversal of the aging process! To prevent or combat chronic inflammation (inflammaging), which can lead to shortening of telomeres, eat an anti-inflammatory diet, control your blood sugar, maintain a healthy weight, and manage stress.

Reversing Hormonal Aging

I was lucky to get through menopause with very few symptoms and I have never taken hormones. However, hormone replacement therapy (HRT) can improve some symptoms of aging (wrinkles, thinning hair, lower sex drive, and lower energy). It may also prevent osteoporosis-related fractures in at-risk women before the age of 60 or within 10 years after menopause. If you are past these stages, or have contraindicating conditions, HRT may not be an option. Do plenty of research and consult with your health care provider.

Lifestyle changes touted for their ability to reverse hormone imbalance naturally include consuming adequate protein and healthy fats such as fatty fish, getting regular exercise, avoiding endocrine disruptors (smoking, pesticides, herbicides, plastics, flame retardants, and fragrances in lotions and cleaning supplies), maintaining a healthy weight, avoiding sugar and refined carbs, managing stress, getting adequate sleep, maintaining healthy gut flora, and drinking green tea (which may help balance insulin). Healthline.com suggests the following supplements as well, but please do your own research before taking any supplement, even natural supplements:

- Nigella seed extract (from the fennel flower), containing thymoquinone, which may mimic estrogen in the body.
- Ashwagandha, aka winter cherry or Indian ginseng, which is an adaptogen believed to help the body overcome stress.
- Black cohosh root, which has historically been used to support women's health issues, including symptoms of menopause; like Nigella seed, it has estrogen-like effects.
- Chasteberry, which may help balance the hormone prolactin, a possible treatment for some PMS symptoms.
- Marjoram, which seems to influence cortisol, estradiol, and insulin.

Intermittent Fasting for Your Health

I'm a fan of intermittent fasting (IF) for its anti-aging and disease prevention benefits. Intermittent fasting is merely delayed eating. By giving our bodies a rest from digestion that extends beyond the nightly sleeping hours, we give them more time to spend on cellular rejuvenation. A 2019 article in the New England Journal of Medicine in 2022 (4) reported two protective benefits of fasting:

- Metabolic switching (As glucose levels decrease, the body switches its energy source from glucose to fat.)
- Cellular stress resistance (Fasting increases resistance to oxidative stress.)

IF triggers multiple changes that slow down aging by keeping cells and DNA healthy :

- **Cellular repair**: IF gives our bodies a chance to remove wastes that would otherwise cause cellular damage.

• **Genetic expression:** Certain genes can be upregulated (expressed) or downregulated (suppressed) through intermittent fasting. According to a 2020 paper from the *Journal of Proteomics*, 30 days of moderate (16:8) intermittent fasting can lead to measurable changes in genes associated with human health and longevity. (5) A 16:8 schedule means 16 hours of not eating and 8 hours of eating. This can be accomplished by ceasing eating at 7 p.m. and not eating again until 11 a.m. the next day.

• **Hormonal changes:** IF drops insulin level, which helps prevents type 2 diabetes.

• **Fights inflammation:** IF decreases inflammation by reducing the number of monocytes in the blood. Monocytes are helpful in fighting infection but an overabundance causes our bodies to think we're under attack, causing an inflammatory response. Our bodies did not evolve to have food available 24-7, and eating without cessation causes an increase in monocytes and inflammation.

• **Protects against oxidative stress:** As mentioned, fasting increases cellular stress resistance. The presence of too many free radicals leads to oxidative stress, which can cause fatigue, muscle and joint pain, memory loss or brain fog, gray hair, decreased eyesight, headaches, wrinkles, susceptibility to infection, and unstable blood sugar levels. IF prevents cellular damage through its seek-and-destroy mission against free radicals.

While restricting eating to between 11 a.m. and 7 p.m. most days can bring about outstanding health and anti-aging benefits, further benefits can be experienced by a full day of fasting once a week or a three-day fast once each month.

Goddess Gift: Inspirational Quotes on Aging

"One day you will look back and see that all along you were blooming." ~ Morgan Harper Nichols

"Anyone who keeps the ability to see beauty never grows old." ~ Franz Kafka

"There is a fountain of youth: it is your mind, your talents, the creativity you bring to your life and the lives of people you love. When you learn to tap this source, you will truly have defeated age." ~ Sophia Loren

"The longer I live, the more beautiful life becomes." ~ Frank Lloyd Wright

"Aging is not lost youth but a new stage of opportunity and strength." ~ Betty Friedan

"Aging is an extraordinary process where you become the person you always should have been." ~ David Bowie

"Know that you are the perfect age. Each year is special and precious, for you shall only live it once." ~ Louise Hay

"I believe the second half of one's life is meant to be better than the first half. The first half is finding out how you do it. And the second half is enjoying it." ~ Frances Lear

"Confidence comes with age, and looking beautiful comes from the confidence someone has in themselves." ~ Kate Winslet

"Getting older makes you more alive. More vitality, more interest, more intelligence, more grace, more expansion." ~ Jamie Lee Curtis

"We have two lives and the second one starts when you realize you only have one." ~ Mario de Elena Andrade-Moon

"As soon as you feel too old to do a thing, DO IT." ~ Margaret Deland

"Act as young as you feel. You're not getting older. You're getting more entitled to be your fabulous self." ~ Gwen Stefani, entertainer

(1) Alan Mozes, "Some People Do Age Faster than Others," HealthDay Reporter, July 6, 2015,
https://www.medicinenet.com/script/main/art.asp?articlekey=189322.

(2) Franceschi, C., and J. Campisi. 2022. "Chronic Inflammation (Inflammaging) And Its Potential Contribution To Age-Associated Diseases". Cited In The National Library Of Medicine.
https://pubmed.ncbi.nlm.nih.gov/24833586/.

(3) Perez, Jason. "NASA's Twins Study Results Published in Science Journal." Text. NASA, September 28, 2018.

http://www.nasa.gov/feature/nasa-s-twins-study-results-published-in-science.

(4) de Cabo, Ph.D., Rafael, and Mark P. Mattson, Ph.D. 2022. "Effects Of Intermittent Fasting On Health, Aging, And Disease | NEJM". New England Journal Of Medicine.

https://www.nejm.org/doi/full/10.1056/NEJMra1905136.

(5) Mindikoglu, Ayse L. 2022. "Intermittent Fasting From Dawn To Sunset For 30 Consecutive Days Is Associated With Anticancer Proteomic Signature And Upregulates Key Regulatory Proteins Of Glucose And Lipid Metabolism, Circadian Clock, DNA Repair, Cytoskeleton Remodeling, Immune System And Cognitive Function In Healthy Subjects". Science Direct.

https://www.sciencedirect.com/science/article/pii/S1874391920300130?fbclid=IwAR3mpd_12xEnTgZhK6LvtkRHB4kTnO_RXQSOMRbyRnr9wksVxd5A4hATF9Q#ec0015.

CHAPTER TWO

GODDESS NUTRITION

FUELING THE GODDESS BODY

Let thy food be thy medicine and medicine be thy food. ~ Hippocrates

Do you ever wonder why there is a "health food" aisle in your local supermarket? Wouldn't it be great if every food item in the store were healthy?

To make their offerings tasty and visually appealing, extend shelf life, and increase profits, food manufacturers add preservatives, flavor enhancers, and dye. The result is that there is little "food" left in our food and some processed foods are at best food-like substances. Worse than "garbage in, garbage out," some of the garbage we eat may establish permanent residence because our bodies don't recognize it and therefore can't process it. To remove the foreign invaders from our bloodstream, our bodies shuttle them off to fat cells. On top of this, because we don't receive adequate nutrition from our food, we aren't satiated and will soon need to eat again. The extra weight we gain and the toxins in overly processed foods cause biological aging.

Processed "Food"

Not all processed food is equal or evil. There's a continuum in food processing, from merely cleaning and removing inedible or unwanted parts to pressing, refining, grinding and milling (used to extract oils from plants, seeds, and nuts or create flour and pasta from whole grains), to foods that have added salt, sugar, or fats (such as canned fruits and vegetables, cheese, freshly made bread, and canned fish), to ultra-processed or highly-processed foods that use artificial colors, flavors, and preservatives to increase shelf life, preserve texture, enhance appearance, and boost flavor.

In some cases, the resulting product from over-processing is little better than poison. For example, in a series of experiments conducted, one group of laboratory rats was fed commercial cereal (e.g., puffed wheat and corn flakes) while another group was fed the boxes the cereal came in. There was more nourishment in the box than in the cereal. (6)

In a very real sense, we are what we eat because what we eat impacts how we feel, look, think, and act. Poor nutrition will result in a weaker body, slower mental processing, less alertness, and a reduced ability to recover from illness and injury. Over time, poor diets can cause high blood pressure, obesity, type 2 diabetes, high cholesterol and heart disease, stroke, gout, cancer, and premature death.

To compensate for nutrient depletion caused by processing, food manufacturers often "enrich" or "fortify" foods, proudly announcing this on their labels, but we should recognize these terms for what they signify: a replacement of nature's nutrients with manufactured ones. Food czars are not gods and they're unable to replicate the healthy nutrition of food in its original form. Nature wins every time.

So, do we all have to eat our food raw? The raw food movement has seen a resurgence in recent years, but most people prefer cooked food. Nutritionists recommend getting as much raw food in our diets as possible, however—particularly leafy greens and every color of the rainbow in vegetables and fruits. A healthy compromise to going 100% raw is to eat a large salad once a day and, for the largest meal of the day, make the plate half vegetables, one-fourth starch, and one-fourth lean protein. Add nuts, seeds, or other healthy fats such as avocado, eggs, or olive oil. Eating healthy fats with your greens boosts their nutrient absorption.

The Gut Biome

The bacteria that live in the gut deserve consideration. Nutritional science is learning that the intestinal microbiome plays a crucial role in reducing the risk of chronic diseases, such as inflammatory bowel disease, obesity, type 2 diabetes, cardiovascular disease, and cancer. A healthy diet contributes to a healthy microbiome, vastly improving our health. The key is to eat a variety of foods and, as Michael Pollan, author of *In Defense of Food*, succinctly states, "Eat food. Not too much. Mostly plants." (7) In addition to their nutritious content, plant foods are high in fiber and stimulate the growth of gut bacteria that feeds on these nutrients. Examples include apples, broccoli, raspberries, artichokes, lentils, green peas, and beans. Other excellent choices are blueberries, pistachios, almonds, and probiotic/fermented foods, such as quality yogurt (avoid the commercial, sweetened kind), kimchi, sauerkraut, kefir, and tempeh. Avoid artificial sweeteners: Aspartame, for instance, is believed to impair insulin response even more than table sugar does. Aspartame has also been linked to disease-causing bacteria associated with gastroenteritis, urinary tract infection, septicemia, meningitis, wound infections, and pneumonia. Aspartame is found in sugar-free sweetener packets, diet soda, gum, low-calorie and no-calorie foods, and some commercial yogurt.

Eating *prebiotic* foods (onions, leeks, asparagus, almonds, garlic, oats, bananas, and chicory) can help the friendly bacteria in our guts produce healthful nutrients.

Inflammation

We talked about inflammation and inflammaging in the last chapter. Inflammation is our body's reaction to stress. This can be from the environment or infection, but it can also come from a poor diet. Adding more veggies, fermented foods, and anti-inflammatory super foods will do wonders for your health. Examples include broccoli, kale, collards, mustard greens, cabbage (especially as sauerkraut), spinach, Swiss chard, beet greens, turnip greens, apple cider vinegar, raw cheese, and kimchi.

Did you know mushrooms feed on dead matter? This speaks to their ability to absorb and eliminate toxins and fight unwanted bacteria and viruses. For this purpose, shitake is one of the best. Maitake (a rare and expensive variety) and Chaga, medicinal mushrooms that have been used for thousands of years, are available as supplements at health food stores, but be sure to research the source. The same is true for cordyceps, which has been linked to longevity, cancer prevention, controlling blood sugar, fat utilization, increasing metabolism, heart health, immune function, and fighting cancer and inflammation.

Anti-inflammatory herbs and spices include ginger, garlic, turmeric, black pepper (freshly ground is best, and when taking turmeric, be sure to take it with black pepper; it can increase curcumin in the turmeric by up to 2,000%), cayenne, cardamom, ginseng, green tea, rosemary, and cinnamon. I used to think Ceylon cinnamon was best, but the most common type, cassia, actually reduces more types of anti-inflammatory markers. Herbs and spices are powerful, so don't overdo them. For instance, you shouldn't take more than one teaspoon of cassia cinnamon per day because excessive amounts can be toxic to the liver.

Alkalinity vs. Acidity

Much of our diet is acidic. Highly acidic foods include sugars and artificial sweeteners, chocolate, wheat bread, white bread, flour and pasta, red meat, beer, eggs, and carbonated soft drinks. Acidic cells lead to chronic pain, impaired metabolism, infections, and cancer. Does this mean you should avoid all acidic foods? No! Many acidic foods are incredibly good for us. But balance is essential because when we eat acid-forming foods our body must counterbalance by releasing alkaline-rich minerals like calcium, phosphorous, and magnesium into our bloodstream. If we're not eating enough alkaline foods, our bodies take these minerals from our bones, teeth, and organs, which can compromise our immune system and make us vulnerable to disease.

The pH scale measures how acidic or alkaline a substance is, and it ranges from 1 (highly acidic) to 14 (highly alkaline). The human body functions best with a pH level as close to 7.4 as possible.

Alkalizing foods include most fruits and vegetables, herbs, nuts, seeds, and herbal teas. Highly alkaline foods include kale, parsley, cucumber, green drinks, broccoli, celery, garlic, spinach, asparagus, green juice (without fruit), Swiss chard, beet greens, sprouts, collard greens, leaf lettuce, mustard greens, salad greens, watercress, cilantro, turmeric, and baking soda, among others. .

To determine your acidic/alkaline balance, you can measure your pH easily at home. Purchase pH strips at the drugstore and measure both urine and saliva pH first thing in the morning. The saliva test tells you your cellular pH and voltage. The urine test gives you your extracellular and lymphatic scores. Both should be in the healthy range, but keep in mind that the pH you measure at home will be 0.8 pH units *below* what is in your body, so you want to aim for a pH of 6.5-7.3.

Below 6.5 is too acidic. Eat fruits and vegetables and raw almonds and take calcium, magnesium, potassium, and zinc. Meditate, reduce stress, and hydrate! Aim to get 80% of your diet from alkalizing food since acid-forming foods are so prevalent in the typical diet. Many people recommend starting your day with a large glass of water with the juice of a whole, freshly-squeezed lemon. Even though lemon is acidic, once it's metabolized by the body, it turns into an alkaline compound about one hour after consuming it. However, this doesn't reduce your body's alkalinity, just that of your urine. This has wonderful protective benefits for your kidneys, but because it can change the alkalinity of your urine, you may get a false pH reading. Just keep that in mind. You may want to test with and without lemon water to see how much of a difference it makes for you. Remember biology class, Goddess? You can use your own body as a test tube!

A pH reading above 7.5 is too alkaline. It's rare to be too alkaline, given that nearly everything the average person consumes, including cooked and processed foods, is acid-forming. If you're testing too alkaline, your body may be in distress from having to call on its "backup system" one too many times to combat poor nutrition. Or you may have very recently ingested a highly alkaline food such as asparagus. If your pH continues to remain highly alkaline, seek medical advice.

Eat the Rainbow

Color signifies nutritional content, and each color has different gifts for the Goddess body.
- **Red** foods, such as apples, cherries, cranberries, radishes, raspberries, red beets, red bell peppers, red-fleshed potatoes, red grapefruit, red onions, strawberries, watermelon, and tomatoes contain beta carotene, quercetin, vitamin A, and lycopene.
- **Orange** foods, such as oranges, orange bell peppers, apricots, butternut and other squashes, tangerines, cantaloupe, mangoes, nectarines, peaches, carrots, persimmons, pumpkin, and sweet potatoes contain beta-carotene, lycopene, and vitamins A & C.
- **Yellow** foods such as bananas, corn, lemons, papaya, pineapple, pomelo, star fruit, yellow beets, yellow bell peppers, yellow grapefruit, and yellow pears contain flavonoids, lycopene, potassium, and beta-carotene. These help build healthy bones, skin, and teeth and improve the heart, digestive, and immune systems.
- **Blue and purple** foods such as blackberries, blueberries, eggplant, plums, purple/red cabbage, purple carrots, purple-fleshed potatoes, and purple grapes contain phytochemicals called anthocyanins, which protect our cardiovascular health and support healthy aging, and resveratrol, known for its anti-aging properties.
- **White** foods such as mushrooms, cauliflower, onions, and garlic contain anthoxanthin and garlic and onion contain allicin, both of which help to lower blood pressure and cholesterol and have anti-inflammatory properties.

Do you have to memorize all of this? Of course not. Just know that each color has a purpose for your good health, so eat the rainbow.

Food's Primary Purpose

The primary purpose of eating and drinking is to nourish and sustain the body, so aim for the following:
- Start each day with a large glass of water. This hydrates the body and replaces fluids lost during sleep.

- Eat a large salad each day with healthy fats (olive oil, nuts, seeds). Make your own dressing from olive oil, balsamic vinegar, or other healthy ingredients. Note that olive oil solidifies when cold, so plan accordingly.
- Grow sprouts. Even if, like me, you're missing a green thumb, it's easy and fun to grow broccoli sprouts. These are nutritional powerhouses, and you can add a handful to your salad or omelet each day. Broccoli sprouts are one of the best. As compared to mature broccoli, broccoli sprouts contain 100 times the amount of sulforaphane, a compound with powerful anti-cancer properties that has 82% bioavailability (meaning its nutritional benefits are easily absorbed). You can find sprouting kits online and at many health food stores, and this is a fun activity to do with children. Mature broccoli is still a superfood though, and contains some health benefits not found in sprouts, so be sure to include both in your diet.
- Avoid overly processed foods.
- Aim for 80% of your food to be raw and/or alkalizing. Get at least five servings of fruits and vegetables every day, emphasizing greens and the rainbow of colors. Include these vegetables as often as possible: broccoli, cabbage, Brussels sprouts, mustard greens, kale, and cauliflower. The next best nutritionally are carrots, onions, beets, spinach; and third, avocadoes, cherries, blackberries, blueberries, raspberries, pineapple, watermelon, kiwi, mangoes, plums, and honeydew melon.
- Drink water throughout the day to stay hydrated. Avoid soda. For a pick-me-up, drink unsweetened tea or coffee (iced or hot).
- Eat healthy fats such as coconut oil, olive oil, and avocado oil. Avoid canola and "vegetable oil," which are rich in omega-6, an overabundance of which causes accelerated growth of cancer cells, blood clotting, and increased bodily inflammation.
- Use real butter, not margarine. Grass-fed is best because it has a greater ratio of healthy unsaturated fats than regular butter and provides vitamin K2, which plays a significant role in bone and heart health.
- Avoid sugar, artificial sweeteners, and sugar substitutes as much as possible. These are toxic to the body. Sugar increases inflammation

and acidity and feeds cancer cells. Agave nectar isn't Goddess food! It contains more fructose than high fructose corn syrup.

- Use alcohol in moderation, if at all. For the Goddess, one drink per day (e.g., five ounces of red wine) is fine.
- Raw nuts are very nutritious, but their skins contain naturally occurring chemicals that can interfere with their nutrient absorption. For optimum nutrition, soak nuts in water for 20 minutes to several hours before consuming. Highest in nutrition are almonds, macadamia nuts, Brazil nuts, and walnuts. Peanuts are not nuts, but legumes, and can be a great source of plant-based protein. However, peanuts contain aflatoxins, which are linked to liver cancer. While commercial peanut butter has lower levels of aflatoxins than freshly ground peanut butter, it should be avoided due to its high sugar content and other additives. Peanuts are also extremely high in omega-6 and low in omega-3. Some alternatives include almond butter, hazelnut butter, macadamia butter, walnut butter, and tahini (sesame seed butter).
- Chew food thoroughly. This increases enzyme production which aids digestion and nutrient absorption.
- Substitute vegetables or a salad for starch (such as potatoes) when eating out.
- Cook vegetables in bone broth rather than water for added nutrition. Bone broth contains collagen and is good for cold, fever, and flu; it improves gut health, strengthens bones, muscles, and tendons, boosts immunity, fortifies nails and hair, reduces inflammation and joint pain, releases toxins, and improves skin elasticity. It's easy to make your own bone broth, but when you buy it from the store, be sure to choose a quality brand, such as Kettle & Fire.
- Buy pasture-raised eggs. Typical supermarket eggs contain only 18 mg of omega-3 (and are high in omega-6), whereas eggs from pasture-raised chickens typically contain 300 mg of omega-3.
- Buy grass-fed organic beef. Cattle raised in feed lots eat grain, and this means they're higher in omega-6. For ethical, environmental, and health reasons, many nutritionists advise using animal protein as a condiment, not as a main meal.

• Eat wild-caught (not farm-raised) fish and shrimp. Around 90% of available shrimp is farm-raised. Farm-raised shrimp often contains antibiotics, and although the US Food and Drug Administration has prohibited their import, it's impossible to be sure that antibiotic-containing shrimp haven't entered the market. Most of the salmon sold at supermarkets and restaurants is farm-raised. Because farm–raised salmon don't eat natural food to provide beneficial antioxidants, their flesh is grey, not pink. To camouflage this unappetizing color, salmon farmers inject their feed with synthetic astaxanthin made from petrochemicals, which turns their flesh bright pink. In addition, farmed salmon live in concentrated pens full of contaminants. Buy wild-caught only. (The package must say "wild.") When dining out, always ask if the salmon you're being served is wild–caught. Don't be fooled by the terms "organic," "imported," or "natural." It must say *wild*.

• Buy organic whenever possible, especially when purchasing the Dirty Dozen, the fruits and vegetables that contain the highest concentrations of pesticides when grown conventionally (see below) and wash fruits and vegetables (even organic ones) before consuming.

The Dirty Dozen

The Environmental Working Group publishes a list of fruits and vegetables to avoid due to their heavy pesticide, chemical, or herbicide use when grown conventionally. This list is called the Dirty Dozen and changes year by year, so be sure to get an updated list. That said, most items on the list are repeat offenders. Buy organic or avoid consuming the following:

1. Strawberries
2. Spinach
3. Kale, collard, and mustard greens
4. Nectarines
5. Apples
6. Grapes (and therefore wine—wine made from organic grapes is available at health food stores and some traditional grocery stores)

7. Cherries
8. Peaches
9. Pears
10. Bell and hot peppers (On some lists, potatoes bumped this one off the Dirty Dozen list; to be safe, buy these organic.)
11. Celery
12. Tomatoes

Clean Up Your Cup of Jo

While not on the Dirty Dozen list, coffee also deserves a mention. I used to buy organic coffee only when it was on sale. Now that I know better, I always buy organic. Conventional coffee is one of the most chemically treated "foods" in the world. The number of pesticides sprayed on coffee far exceeds those used on the Dirty Dozen. It's also steeped in herbicides, synthetic fertilizers, fungicides, and insecticides. These are bad for the environment and bad for you. Brazil, which is the world's leading coffee growing region, increased its usage of chemicals used on conventionally grown coffee by 800% from 1990 levels.

Less than 10% of available coffee is grown organically. Choose that.

The Clean 15

To save on your grocery bill, you can take heart in the fact that there is also a Clean 15 list of fruits and vegetables that can safely be purchased in their non-organic version.

1. Avocados
2. Sweet corn (but buy organic if you can't find non-GMO options)
3. Pineapple
4. Frozen sweet peas
5. Onions
6. Papaya (but buy organic if you can't find non-GMO options)
7. Eggplant
8. Asparagus
9. Kiwi
10. Cabbage

11. Cauliflower
12. Cantaloupes
13. Broccoli
14. Mushrooms
15. Honeydew melons

To be honest, except for avocadoes (which are expensive) I almost always buy the Clean 15 in their organic versions. It's just too much bother to try to remember which are safe to eat in their non-organic version. An added benefit is supporting organic farming, which is better for the environment.

About Supplements

Given the factors associated with aging and the deteriorating nutrition in our food, supplementation is often necessary. I'm not consistent with my supplementation regimen, but I do take a multivitamin, collagen, and a probiotic regularly. In addition, I often take vitamins C, E, and D, fish oil, calcium/magnesium, aloe vera gel, and co-enzyme Q10.

The National Institute of Health says that while not everyone needs supplements, they can be useful for filling nutritional gaps. All vitamins and minerals have a safe upper limit, so try not to get too much of a good thing. If you're already getting adequate amounts of a vitamin or mineral in your food or in a multivitamin (with the possible exception of vitamin C, which is difficult to overdo), there's no need to supplement further. And make sure any supplements you do take come from a quality manufacturer that uses third-party testing.

The following are supplements to consider:

- A **multivitamin** (Aim for food-based ones, which won't hurt your stomach if taken without food.)
- **Calcium:** Women age 19-50 need 1,000 mg/daily; 51 and older women need 1,200 mg/daily.
- **B12** vitamins (present in meat, fish, and dairy), 2.4 mcg/daily.
- **Vitamin C:** Your body can only absorb only about 400 mg at a time, so make sure you get it throughout the day. Up to 2,000 mg is recommended, but those with kidney disease, liver disease, or

gout should limit their daily intake to 1,000 mg or check with their medical provider.

- **Vitamin D**: Most of us are vitamin D deficient, so supplementing with 2,000-4,000 IU daily is optimal. You can get a good dose by spending 10-30 minutes in the sun at midday provided enough skin is exposed.
- **Co-enzyme Q10**: A deficiency of this is linked to mitochondrial conditions, cardiac disease, strokes, and neurodegenerative diseases such as Alzheimer's disease and Parkinson's. Deficiency has also been linked to the fragility common in aging. A 2018 University of Colorado Boulder study published by the American Heart Association found significant health benefits of taking 20 milligrams of Q10 a day for participants 60 years of age and older. (8)
- **Probiotics**: These help maintain good gut health, which is vital to nutrient absorption and disease prevention. Benefits are strain-specific. The most common probiotics are lactobacilli and bifidobacteria. If you're overwhelmed by the choices, consult a nutritionist or opt for other routes to a healthy gut, including a healthy diet that incorporates fermented foods and daily exercise.
- **Fish oil**: Fish oil supplements can augment your omega-3 consumption. It's generally safe to take up to 3 grams of quality fish oil daily in supplement form.
- **Vitamin E**: Vitamin E helps support healthy vision and the health of your blood, brain, and skin. It also has antioxidant properties. Deficiency in vitamin E can cause nerve pain (neuropathy). The recommended daily amount for adults is 15 mg/day. If you already get this in your multivitamin, you're good.

Goddess Gift: The Salad Hack

If you struggle to get a daily salad into your diet because of the hassle of preparing it, there are some delicious bagged salad kits available. However, few of them are organic, and both spinach and kale are on the "Dirty Dozen" and should only be purchased organically. If you can find organic bagged salad kits, stock up for the week! Or try my economical salad hack: Each week prepare a large "basic" green salad (enough for the week) with greens, sliced radishes, sliced peppers, and sprouts and place it in an air-tight container in the refrigerator. Take out enough for one meal and add the goodies: cheese, nuts or seeds, dried berries, apple cubes, mandarin sections, or other fruits and veggies. In this way, you can have a different salad each day with very little prep work. You can turn your salad into a main dish by adding smoked salmon or cooked chicken. Or make it into a taco salad with seasoned beef, a few crumbled tortilla chips, shredded cheese, and salsa.

Keep in mind that most commercial salad dressings are loaded with ingredients not fit for the Goddess body (yes, even some that call themselves Green Goddess!), so check the ingredients or make your own. A simple balsamic dressing with a quality balsamic vinegar, garlic powder, black pepper, and olive oil takes just a minute to make. Add a squeeze of lemon juice and you'll never go back to commercial dressings again.

(6) "Breakfast Cereals And The Rat Experiments - Craig Eymann Chiropractic". 2022. Craig Eymann Chiropractic. http://drcraig.chiro dev2.com/breakfast-cereals-and-the-rat-experiments/.

(7) Pollan, Michael. 2009. In Defense Of Food. Turtleback Books.

(8) Marshall, Lisa. 2022. "Novel Antioxidant Makes Old Blood Vessels Seem Young Again". CU Boulder Today. https://www.colorado.edu/today/2018/04/19/novel-antioxidant-makes-old-blood-vessels-seem-young-again.

CHAPTER THREE
GODDESSES DETOX

CONQUERING HIDDEN ENEMIES

The accumulation of toxins ... accelerates aging. The elimination of toxins awakens the capacity for renewal. ~ Deepak Chopra

Aging results from cellular damage, and cellular damage occurs for two reasons: *deficiency* and *toxicity*. In the last chapter, we talked about getting adequate nutrients. Fueling our body with appropriate nutrition is the primary way to guard against cellular *deficiency*. In this chapter, we'll look at how to prevent cellular *toxicity*: what toxins are, where they come from, how to avoid them, and how to get rid of them.

Strictly speaking, a *toxin* is a poisonous substance produced by plants, animals, or microorganisms, such as the bacterium that causes botulism. But when most people talk about toxins, they're referring to any compound that can harm health. Under that definition, toxins are in the air we breathe, the water we drink, the food we eat, the cleansers we use, and the lotions and potions we slather on our bodies. The European Chemicals agency estimates that there are more than 144,000 human-made chemicals in existence, (9) and the Centers for Disease Control and Prevention (CDC) has measured more than

400 environmental chemicals in human urine, blood, serum, breast milk, and meconium. (10) The Global Alliance on Health and Pollution estimates that toxic pollutants are responsible for 15 percent of all premature deaths worldwide. (11) Even when they don't kill, toxins can significantly impair our health and the quality of our lives.

Many toxins have endocrine-disrupting properties that bond with hormone receptors and mimic hormones. Breast cancer and prostate cancer are two diseases caused by the dysregulation of hormone systems. Endocrine disruptors can also slow thyroid function, which reduces metabolism and increases the risk of obesity. Our bodies have natural detoxification abilities, but we haven't evolved enough to combat all the toxins now prevalent in our environment. Toxins can overload detoxification pathways in our liver and block enzymes that burn fat, increasing our risk for cancer, fatty liver, and other diseases.

Exacerbating the toxic problem, we thwart our body's natural detoxification processes (sweat, urination, and breathing) by wearing antiperspirants, not getting adequate exercise, not drinking enough water, and not getting enough fresh air.

When the body encounters a toxin, it shuttles it off into fat cells (adipose tissue) to keep it from harming our organs and other tissues. However, overaccumulation of toxins can easily overload the system. While we shouldn't wait for symptoms to appear, obvious symptoms of toxic overload include acne (outside of the teen years), rashes, a pot belly, dark circles under our eyes, body odor, thyroid issues, allergies, and congestion.

Following are some common toxins and toxin-containing products we should strive to reduce or eliminate.

Fluoride, Arsenic, and Chlorine

As we've discussed, one reason adults get cancer is a decline in the body's ability to repair damaged DNA. Fluoride, which is added to 60% of the tap water in the U.S., has been shown to disrupt DNA repair enzymes. At high doses, fluoride can actually damage people's teeth, according to the World Health Organization, (12) and some research links it to more serious side effects, including bone cancer and cognitive impairments. From 2009-2019, more than 300 municipalities in North America voted to end fluoridation programs over health concerns. (13) In Europe, most countries do not fluoridate, and those that do limit its use (Poland, for instance, only fluoridates 1% of its water). The only exception is Ireland, which fluoridates 73% of its water. (14)

Fluoride is present in most toothpaste due to its "cavity fighting" benefits. However, its ability to prevent cavities is suspect because cavity rates have declined similarly across fluoridated and non-fluoridated communities and municipalities with fluoridated water often have higher cavity rates than those that don't. (15) If your community fluoridates water (and even if it doesn't) consider using a multi-step filtering system to remove the fluoride. We use a Berkey filter (bigberkeywaterfilters.com) to make sure our water is free from contaminants, even though our municipality doesn't fluoridate. We use it to purify not only drinking water but also our cooking water. When there was a "boil order" due to contamination entering our public water system, our filtered water was still safe to drink. Whatever filtration system you use, make sure it removes bacteria, such as E. coli, chlorine, heavy metals, volatile organic compounds, and pharmaceuticals. Most water filters you can purchase in grocery and department stores are inadequate for this task. A friend who had a health scare first filters her water with a grocery store filter, then uses that water to fill her Big Berkey. Beware of too much of a good thing, however: over filtering can strip essential minerals that are naturally present in water.

Consumer Reports has found that the water purification systems in many communities haven't kept pace with the increasing levels of pollution in the environment. (16) We need look no further than the tragedy of Flint, Michigan, to see that we can't take our water safety for granted.

Arsenic is in most fluoridated water and has been linked to depression, high blood pressure, and circulatory problems. Arsenic is also present in brown rice and brown rice syrup! It exists on the outside of rice; this shell is removed to make white rice. If you eat a lot of rice, consider switching to white rice, and eating less rice overall. Rice is the biggest food source of inorganic arsenic, a more toxic form of arsenic. Also limit consumption of products that contain rice, such as rice milk, rice bran, rice cereal, rice crackers, and cereal bars containing rice and/or brown rice syrup.

Chlorine is often present in drinking water, even when fluoride isn't. Chlorine enters the body as a result of breathing, swallowing, or skin contact, and it reacts with phenol in water to produce acids. These acids are corrosive, and high levels of chlorine damage cells in the body on contact. Long-term exposure to chemicals in drinking water can cause cancer. Yet in the U.S., it's added to our drinking water as a disinfectant. European countries don't use chlorine in their water.

Even when you filter your drinking and cooking water, you're exposed to the chemicals in your municipal water when bathing and showering. Exposure to vaporized chlorine (such as steam in the shower) is 100 times more damaging than drinking chlorinated water. Consider installing a showerhead filter. A more expensive solution is a whole-house filtration system, which may be worth it for your peace of mind and would eliminate the need for a separate water filter. At a minimum, filter your drinking and cooking water (including the water you use to make coffee or tea).

Plastic Water Bottles

Carry water in glass water bottles, not plastic. Americans drink more bottled water than we do coffee, tea, milk, soft drinks, or any other beverage, most of it from plastic bottles. While drinking more water is a good thing, *Consumer Reports* tested 47 popular bottled waters (35 noncarbonated, 12 carbonated) and found toxic levels of per- and poly-fluoroalkyl substances (PFAS) chemicals, which have been linked to health issues across the immunological, developmental and reproductive, hepatic, hormonal, and carcinogenic spectrum. (17) Toxicity level varied among bottlers, but how much toxicity is acceptable?

I don't drink bottled water or carbonated beverages from plastic. Plastic often contains Bisphenol A (BPA), known for health risks such as hormone disruption and genetic damage. When the public became aware of the health risks of BPA, many manufacturers switched to alternatives. However, the most common substitute (Bisphenol S, or

BPS) is equally harmful. "BPA-free" on a label often means it uses BPS. These bisphenols are also used to line aluminum cans used for storing vegetables, soups, and beans, among others.

Plastic packaging can leach toxins, especially polyvinyl chloride (PVC) into our food. Never microwave or otherwise heat food in plastic. If you choose to use plastic wrap to keep food fresh, wrap it first in non-bleached parchment paper so the plastic doesn't come into contact with the food, or use alternatives such as glass storage containers or beeswax wraps, available at health food stores and online sites. Other options include silicone lids and bowl covers. Look for those that are 100% food grade, lead-free, BPA- and BPS-free, phthalate-free, PVC-free, and non-toxic. It's a lot to remember. Research first, purchase second.

K-Cups and Other Single-Use Coffee Capsules

I used to have a codependent relationship with my Nespresso machine. I loved my beans! I would have several cups of espresso a day (darker beans actually have less caffeine, so no, I wasn't walking on the ceiling). I loved the convenience of just popping in a pod, pressing a lever, and having a lovely cup of espresso in a minute or two. At some point, it occurred to me that shooting piping hot water through aluminum and plastic, and then drinking the end product wasn't healthy. After some research, I learned that coffee brewed from capsule machines can contain estrogenic chemicals that migrate from the plastic, which can mess with our hormonal system. And aluminum exposure (pods are also made with aluminum) has been linked to Alzheimer's, depression, anxiety, and autoimmune disease. (18) A study at the University of Barcelona found that pod coffee contains five times the amount of toxins present in instant or drip coffee, including furan, a chemical that's been shown to be carcinogenic in animals. (19) It's still within "safety levels" unless you drink an unusual amount of coffee each day. However, if you're trying to limit your exposure to toxins, this is a pretty easy source to eliminate.

Thinking about what my several-times daily fixes might be doing to my body over time took the joy out of it, so I gave up my machine. Instead, I buy organic espresso and brew it in an old-school stainless steel espresso pot on the stove. While it's not as convenient, I have come to enjoy the ritual of filling the pot with water, spooning in the espresso, tamping it down, and listening for the bubbling that signals it's ready.

Single-use coffee capsules are also an environmental concern. Keurig Green Mountain sold 13.2 billion capsules in 2018. By 2012, Nespresso had sold 27 billion worldwide. Nearly half (41%) of U.S. households use single-serve brewing systems in their homes. (20) These end up in landfills because recycling requires separating the materials (so much for the convenience factor), and even then, many municipalities don't recycle the type of plastic they use. Nespresso has a ship-back-for-free option, but it requires drop-off and isn't available in many areas. Estimates are that very few capsules are recycled.

Fortunately, new products are being developed to address the environmental concern. One example is WayCap, a stainless steel and silicone pod that's fillable and reusable and compatible with Nespresso machines. There is also a stainless steel K-Cup available (make sure to choose the one not made with plastic). These are not only environmentally friendly and healthier, but also far less expensive than single-use capsules. Just be sure to choose organic coffee, as mentioned in the previous chapter.

Aluminum

Aluminum in the bloodstream has the ability to bypass the blood-brain barrier and enter the brain. Therefore, as cited earlier, its toxicity is associated with neurodegenerative diseases, such as Parkinson's, dementia, and Alzheimer's. Aluminum is commonly included in vaccines, such as the flu vaccine, for its ability to trigger a bodily reaction that increases the uptake of the vaccine. Aluminum hampers the body's ability to use calcium, magnesium, phosphorous, and vitamin A, setting us up for osteoporosis.

Many of us put aluminum under our arms every day, sometimes several times a day, often right after shaving. Aluminum chloralhydrate salts in antiperspirants work by dissolving on skin and melting into pores, plugging the pores, and preventing sweat. But sweat is part of our body's natural detoxification system. It's healthy to sweat, but it doesn't mean we have to stink. Swap antiperspirant for a non-aluminum containing *deodorant* instead.

Another issue with aluminum salts is that they can collect in breast tissue. Although inconclusive, some studies suggest that aluminum chloralhydrate salts are a causative factor in breast cancer.

Our kidneys are part of our detoxification system and useful in eliminating aluminum. Because of this, the National Kidney Foundation advises patients with advanced kidney disease against using skin care products containing aluminum. Kidneys that already work at suboptimum levels can't clear out aluminum fast enough. But shouldn't the rest of us also protect our kidneys as much as possible? Why make them work harder to eliminate something we can simply avoid?

After trying several brands of aluminum-free deodorant, I've settled on the Humble brand, a natural deodorant. I find that it's perfect for combatting odor and I don't have to reapply it during the day as I used to with other natural brands. Like me, you may have to test a few brands to find one that works for you.

Aluminum has been linked to chronic kidney disease and dementia, rheumatism, and migraines, but researchers found that most of those afflicted with these conditions got their high aluminum levels from medications, not antiperspirants. Aluminum hydroxide is used in medications for heartburn relief, sour stomach, and peptic ulcer pain. Brand names that at present contain aluminum hydroxide include Mylanta, Maalox, and Gaviscon. Antacids and buffered aspirin contain aluminum as well. Pregnant women should avoid over-the-counter antacids that contain aluminum because these can act as powerful neurological toxins in utero.

If you choose to use aluminum foil in cooking, first wrap your food in natural (non-bleached) parchment paper to avoid your food coming into contact with aluminum. Choose non-aluminum cookware (such as ceramic, ceramic-enameled, glass, or cast iron). If you use cast iron, you may want to take an iron-free multivitamin because you'll likely get iron in your food when cooking.

Mercury

Mercury exposure is harmful to adults and children and is especially damaging when exposure occurs in vitro. Mercury in adults can cause fatigue, weakness, irritability, loss of memory and coordination, tremors, and hearing and vision problems, and numbness, burning, or tingling of lips, fingers, and toes. High levels of mercury can damage the brain and kidneys and cause circulatory failure.

Mercury is present in nearly all bodies of water due to industrial discharge. Because it binds to protein, it's also present in all fish and shellfish to some degree. Advisories to limit consumption of fish and shellfish from freshwater and coastal areas have been issued in all 50 states in the U.S., Nineteen states have also issued advisories regarding fish-containing mercury in their coastal waters. (21) The greatest concentration of mercury in fish has been found in larger fish, such as halibut, tuna, and swordfish. Even though I love all three of these, I limit my consumption to rare occasions. If you eat tuna, avoid white tuna (albacore) because its mercury levels are three times higher than the smaller skipjack tuna. "Canned light" is safer than albacore, but avoid "gourmet" and "tonno" varieties, which are made with larger yellowfin tuna and contain mercury levels on par with those of albacore.

Mercury has also been used in dental amalgams (mistakenly called "silver" fillings) for the past 150 years. In addition to being an environmental hazard, amalgams leak, and mercury-containing fillings can break off and be swallowed. In both cases, this introduces mercury into our bloodstream. Chewing and drinking hot liquids can also release mercury from fillings into the bloodstream. As of 2020, the FDA has recommended against the use of mercury for dental fillings for "high-risk populations," but some dentists continue to use them. If you already have amalgam fillings, it's generally not recommended to remove them unless there's decay beneath them or they are worn or cracked, because the removal process can increase the risk of accidental swallowing. If you do decide to remove them for any reason, research the safety procedures and experience of the dentist you use. Look for a holistic dentist experienced in the safe removal of amalgams.

Mercury is also present in hemorrhoidal cream that contains shark liver oil, in some contact lens solutions, in certain diuretics, and in vaccines containing the ingredient thimerosal, which is 49% mercury by weight. Even though for decades thimerosal was touted as safe to add to vaccines, public outcry has resulted in it being eliminated from most childhood vaccines. It may still be present in limited amounts in some and it's still used as a preservative in the multi-dose flu vaccine. Always ask to see the package insert and research the ingredients of any vaccine you choose to accept.

Radon

Radon is the off-gassing of uranium decay present in the soil. Colorless and odorless, radon is the number one cause of lung cancer in non-smokers, killing 21,000 people annually in the US and EU. (22) Although it's everywhere, even in the air we breathe, levels vary dramatically. Certain areas of the country are known for being radon "hot spots," but elevated levels can exist anywhere. Homes right next to one another can have vastly different radon levels. The only way to know for sure is to test.

The EPA recommends every homeowner test for radon annually because radon levels can change over time. The picocurie per liter (pCi/L) unit of measurement is used in the US. Most countries that use the metric system, as well as the World Health Organization (WHO), measure in becquerels per cubic meter; 1 pCi/L is equal to 37 Bq/m3. The best radon level is zero, but that's an impossibility. For every 2.7 pCi/L, (99.9 Bq/m3), lung cancer risks rise by 16%. WHO recommends mitigation for levels above 2.7 pCi/L (the EPA's action level is 4 pCi/L) or 100 Bq/m3. What you don't know can hurt you, so it's best to test. The good news is, if elevated radon levels are found, mitigation systems are easy and inexpensive to install, and they can drop radon down to safer levels in just a day or two. Passive home testing kits are available at hardware stores for around $15 plus $40 for lab fees. Active radon testing requires power and provides hourly readings, then calculates an average level over the testing period. Radon testing technicians charge approximately $125 to $150 to place and pick up the testing equipment and provide your results.

Mold

Exposure to high levels of mold is a health hazard and is particularly dangerous for those with breathing difficulties. I once toured a home that had been shut up for several years. The electricity and heat were disconnected, so we had to use a flashlight to navigate the hallways. Breathing became difficult, and it wasn't until we got back outside that I began to realize just how bad the air had been. The home had a mold issue—black mold. I had chest pain and breathing issues for two days after that visit. Regular household mold can cause congestion problems and allergic reactions similar to hay fever. Molds produce spores, which drift through the air, and like radon, they're present in all indoor environments. The EPA recommends humidity levels of below 60% to prevent mold accumulation. Running a dehumidifier to reduce indoor moisture, leaving windows open for air circulation, using fans when cooking, and cleaning regularly can prevent toxic mold accumulation in the home. To clean mold, wipe with a solution of soap and water or a diluted bleach solution. Dry the surface well after cleaning.

Mildew is a precursor to mold. It's often gray, black, brown, or white and appears as a powdery substance on the surface of a wall or ceiling in a moist area, such as a bathroom. It is easily wiped off.

Toxins in Our Food

Pesticides are a toxin in our food that we discussed in the previous chapter. To reduce your risk of pesticide exposure from food, eat organic as often as possible, especially when it comes to the Dirty Dozen. Avoid adding toxins to your food via aluminum or plastic. Avoid contact with these materials by wrapping food first in natural parchment paper.

It's a controversial choice, but I've read enough to decide that a microwave has no place in our family's kitchen. Do your own research. Some studies have shown that amino acids change shape during microwave cooking, rendering them unusable to the human body. Other studies disagree. If you choose to use a microwave (as so many do), always use microwave-safe cooking containers.

Cadmium, found in some chocolate, cigarettes, vapes, nori (edible seaweed), and metal containers, has been classified by the International Agency for Research on Cancer as a human carcinogen linked to increased cancer risk. (23) Dark chocolate had levels one-tenth of that found in cocoa powders. The EU has set limits on the amount of cadmium that may be present in chocolate; the U.S. has no such limits, but California does require a warning label on products that have more than 4.1 mg of cadmium per daily serving.

Carrageenan, used as a stabilizer in foods such as almond milk, can cause gastrointestinal inflammation and disease and can lead to chronic illnesses such as diabetes, digestive disorders, cardiovascular disease, neurological disorders, and cancer. Carrageenan is even present in some organic foods. It's commonly found in non-organic products, such as rotisserie chicken, deli meats, dairy, and other processed foods.

Lead is detrimental to our brain, liver, kidneys, and bones, and can cause cognitive issues, osteoporosis, hearing loss, and hypertension. Lead is present in our drinking water, some imported glazed pottery, vintage dishware, and many dietary supplements. Lead is also present in some chocolate. No level of lead is considered safe, but the Food and Drug Administration allows as much as 0.1 ppm of lead in candy consumed by young children. Why is any amount of lead allowed in candy consumed by children given how detrimental lead is to a child's brain development? The agencies established to protect us (the EPA, the FTC, the FDA, the CDC, and the WHO) are subject to multiple pressures and fierce lobbying (industrial, societal, economic, and political). Therefore, we should consider any of their recommendations to be the bare minimum of safety levels and do our best to protect our health well beyond these levels.

Glutamates are produced in the body and are present in many foods naturally, such as parmesan and Roquefort cheeses, Asian sauces (soy, fish, oyster), nuts, cured ham, fresh tomatoes, grape juice, seafood, mushrooms, peas, and starchy vegetables. However, using glutamate as an additive (as it is in many processed foods) isn't advised because of the health risks associated with its consumption, including headaches, heart palpitations, brain cell injury, cellular inflammation, and liver damage. Glutamate is added to many processed foods disguised as ingredients such as natural flavors, spices, hydrolyzed protein, hydrolyzed yeast, soy extract, yeast extract, autolyzed yeast, protein isolate, vegetable protein, sodium caseinate, textured protein, and soy protein extract. Even restaurants that advertise no **MSG (monosodium glutamate)** on their menus likely include it. MSG has been linked to obesity, metabolic disorders, brain toxicity, reduced pain sensitivity, anxiety, depression, stress, and temporary spikes in blood pressure.

Genetically modified organisms (GMOs) have been called "mad science" by some and are outlawed in many countries around the world. In the laboratory, GMOs have been shown to shorten the lifespan and increase tumors in rats, and cause liver and kidney damage. In humans, GMOs have led to allergic and inflammatory responses and have been linked to arthritis, multiple sclerosis, and irritable bowel disease. GMOs are present in non-organically produced corn, soybeans, canola oil, cottonseed oil, sugar beets, papayas grown in Hawaii, popcorn, soy sauce, frozen pizza, frozen dinners, dry cereal, baby formula, canned soups, cookies, and ice cream. In several states, including my home state of Oregon, health advocates have pressed for GMO warning labels. Until that occurs, look for foods labeled "non GMO" and foods certified organic. By law, these can't introduce GMOs into the food and must be processed without artificial ingredients, pesticides, or fertilizer, but even organic corn and soy have likely been cross-contaminated. It may be wise to limit corn and soy consumption (and when you do buy it, choose organic).

Glyphosate is the active ingredient in Roundup, a ubiquitous and toxic herbicide used on crops and plants to kill weeds. The WHO has classified glyphosate as "probably carcinogenic to humans." (24) Glyphosate has made it into our food supply on produce, in meat from animals that consume plants sprayed by the herbicide, and in packaged foods. While you can't eliminate it entirely, you can drastically reduce your exposure to glyphosate by eating organic fruits, vegetables, and protein (meat and collagen should come from 100% grass-fed cows). If you consume a lot of glyphosate-rich foods, some health advisors recommend supplementing with 3,000 mg of glycine daily to help offset glyphosate toxicity. Glycine is often found in collagen products, so if you take collagen, it may offer you some protection.

Toxins in the Air We Breathe

Volatile organic compounds (VOCs) are compounds that easily enter the air through their high vapor pressure and have low water solubility. Many VOCs are human-made chemicals. You've probably seen paint advertised as "low VOC" or "no VOC." This refers to the presence or absence of these compounds, but don't be fooled. When it comes to indoor air quality, the definition under the Clean Air Act for a VOC refers to its photochemical reactivity. That means that some products that are labeled as "low VOC" or "no VOC" under the Clean Air Act may actually be highly toxic. According to the EPA website:

> "While it is prudent to use products with lower VOC levels, it does not assure that the products are any better (and they may even be worse) than products with higher VOCs. (25)

VOCs can have both short- and long-term health effects and are often present indoors at high concentrations. They're found in cleaning products, pesticides, building materials and furnishings, office equipment (such as copiers and printers), craft materials such as glue and adhesive, permanent markers, and photographic solutions. Can you smell it? It's likely a VOC.

So, what's a Goddess to do? Use natural cleaning products and natural scents whenever possible. Toxin-free cleaning products include lemon juice, baking soda, white vinegar, rubbing alcohol, and Borax. At minimum, purchase unscented products and avoid artificial air fresheners. And introduce plenty of fresh air into your home.

Skin Care, Beauty Products, Personal Products

The beauty and personal care industries are virtually unregulated. This frequently leads to the presence of untested chemicals in their products.

While a one-time exposure to a toxin may not cause harm, toxins have a cumulative effect and may cause actual harm when combined with other chemicals.

Toxic chemicals to avoid in skin care and beauty products include formaldehyde (a known carcinogen) and its kissing cousins, paraformaldehyde, methylene glycol, and quaternium 15 (it releases formaldehyde), mercury, dibutyl and diethylhexyl phthalates (hormone and endocrine disrupters), isobutyl and isopropyl parabens (hormone disrupter), polyfluoroalkyl substances (PFAS), linked to cancer, and m- and o-phenylenediamine, used in hair dyes, which can cause DNA damage and cancer. Also avoid BHA and BHT, coal tar dyes, DEA-related ingredients, parabens, petrolatum, polyethylene glycol (PEGS) sometimes seen as ceteareth in deodorant, makeup, styling gel, and shaving cream, siloxanes, sodium lareth sulfate and sodium lauryl sulphate (common in shampoos), and triclosan (used in some antiperspirants and deodorants, cleansers, and hand sanitizers). Also avoid fragrances, which may combine hundreds of undisclosed chemicals.

Sunscreen can protect from the damaging effects of the sun's rays, but some ingredients may cause damage of their own. Avoid sunscreen containing oxybenzone (benzophenone-3), which is classified as a hazardous irritant for the eyes and slightly hazardous for direct skin contact. When exposing your skin to the sun for a limited time, try coconut oil instead of sunscreen (it has a natural SPF level of between 6 and 8) and remember that sunshine is nature's vitamin D. A little sun exposure (without overdoing it) is healthy.

Detoxing Naturally

Natural forms of detoxification include exercise to the point of sweating, saunas, and eating cruciferous vegetables (cauliflower, broccoli, cabbage) and probiotic foods (e.g., kefir, sauerkraut). Need another reason to eat your leafy greens? Chlorophyll, the green pigment in green leafy vegetables, can bind with many toxic substances and remove them from the body when eliminating.

Houseplants, especially cactus, snake plants, spider plants, aloe vera, ivy, asparagus fern, and rubber plants, help remove many toxic and cancer-causing VOC from our indoor air (e.g., formaldehyde and benzene). So do HEPA filters and HEPA vacuum cleaners. A 1989 NASA study (26) found that placing at least two large plants for every 100 square feet (9.3 square meters) is optimum for detoxifying the air, and the bigger and leafier, the better. Other studies recommend 10 plants per small room and 16-32 plants for large rooms (yes, you'd have your own nursery at this point!). Larger pots are best to expose the surface of the soil because bacteria and fungi in the soil use the broken-down toxins, aiding air purification.

Moving your lymph nodes daily is also an important way to detoxify. Just 30 minutes of walking or five minutes bouncing on a mini trampoline is enough to get your lymph moving.

Other ways to detoxify include staying hydrated, dry brushing your skin, stretching (e.g., yoga), fortifying with vitamin C and green tea extract, and intermittent fasting.

Intermittent Fasting for Detox

I love **intermittent fasting** (IF) so much that I authored *Goddesses Don't Diet: The Girlfriends' Guide to Intermittent Fasting*. We've already discussed IF's anti-aging and disease prevention benefits, but fasting even for short periods (such as postponing your first meal of the day, and not eating after dinner) also has outstanding detoxifying benefits. The body uses a lot of energy to digest food. When fasting, energy normally used by the digestive system can be used for metabolism and restoration of the immune system. The body uses that energy to search for dead cells, damaged tissues, fatty deposits, tumors, and abscesses, and it takes them apart, burning them for fuel, or expelling them as waste. During fasting, the body also rebuilds damaged tissues. In *The Anti-Aging Plan*, author Dr. Roy Walford recommends fasting one day a week or three to four days in a row once a month. IF and extended fasting have been linked in many studies for cancer prevention benefits. (27) I've done several multi-day fasts including one 14-day challenge while writing *Goddesses Don't Diet*. In the book,

I shared my phenomenal before and after lab results for blood sugar levels, triglycerides, cholesterol, and more.

In short, fasting has health benefits far beyond weight loss. The Massachusetts Institute of Technology reports that this single dietary change is enough to reverse age-related stem cell decline. (28)

Other Ways to Detox

Colon cleanses, chelation therapy, and coffee enemas are aggressive methods of detox that may remove beneficial bacteria as well. Use these with caution, because these may remove toxins from fat cells (where our bodies store toxins safely out of the way) only to disperse them throughout other parts of the body. If you use these methods, work with a knowledgeable practitioner and take activated charcoal. Activated charcoal will grab hold of the toxins pulled from fat cells to help keep them from entering other body systems. Activated charcoal is fine to take in any case. It has been linked to longevity although high doses can cause constipation and it should be taken separately from other medicines and supplements because of its clear-the-deck properties.

More Detox Tips

WebDetoxMeApp.org is a great place for tips and up-to-date news on detoxing your lifestyle. Here are a few tips from that site that we haven't already covered.

- Don't buy antibacterial dish soap. (The site also cautions against antibacterial hand and body soap.)
- Wash new clothes at least once before wearing.
- Choose a quick-drying cloth, such as nylon, instead of vinyl shower curtains. Avoid buying clothing and other accessories made from vinyl.
- Avoid toothpaste containing triclosan.
- Avoid dry cleaning; instead, find a professional wet cleaner or laundry service.
- Avoid commercial dryer sheets. Instead, use a wool dryer ball to soften clothes in the dryer.

- Wash your hands after you clean out the lint in the dryer.
- If you must purchase items in plastic, choose recycle numbers 1, 2, 4, or 5 instead of 3, 6, or 7.
- Open your windows periodically to air out your home.
- Avoid chlorine bleach or bleach products for everyday cleaning.
- Remove skin and fat from meat and fish before consuming.
- Buy pajamas without flame-resistant chemicals.
- Don't use mothballs.
- Keep dust low by using a clean damp cloth (or microfiber).

Another great resource to consider is the book, *Toxic Relief: Restore Health and Energy through Fasting and Detoxification*, by Don Colbert, M.D.

Goddess Gift: How to Boost Glutathione

Glutathione is a potent antioxidant naturally produced in the body. Dr. Mark Hyman, author of *10-Day Detox Diet*, calls glutathione the most critical part of our bodies' detoxification system. Toxins stick to glutathione, and it carries them out of our bodies through our elimination process. Oral supplementation with glutathione has mixed results, so here are **10 ways to boost your glutathione levels naturally**:

1. Eat glutathione-rich foods. These include spinach, avocados, asparagus, and okra.

2. Eat sulfur-rich foods: beef, fish, poultry, broccoli, Brussel sprouts, cauliflower, kale, watercress, mustard greens, garlic, shallots, and onions.

3. Get added vitamin C through citrus fruits, broccoli, kiwi, bell peppers, and papaya. Consider supplementing with 500-1,000 mg of vitamin C. Studies have found that regular supplementation with vitamin C can boost glutathione levels in blood cells.

4. Add selenium, which boosts glutathione. Selenium-rich foods include Brazil nuts, chicken, beef, fish, cottage cheese, and organ meats.

5. Add whey protein, which contains cysteine, an amino acid that helps synthesize glutathione.

6. Consider supplementing with milk thistle, which can increase glutathione levels.

7. Consider supplementing with turmeric for its curcumin content. Turmeric can increase glutathione levels, and turmeric extract provides a concentrated boost.

8. Sleep well. Lack of sleep can decrease glutathione levels.

9. Exercise regularly, which can help maintain glutathione levels.

10. Limit alcohol. Excess alcohol consumption reduces glutathione levels in the lungs.

(9) Scientists Categorize Earth As A 'Toxic Planet'". 2022. Phys.Org. https://phys.org/news/2017-02-scientists-categorize-earth-toxic-planet.html.

(10) "Environmental Chemicals". 2022. Centers for Disease Control and Prevention.

(10) "Environmental Chemicals". 2022. Centers for Disease Control and Prevention. https://www.cdc.gov/biomonitoring/environmental_ chemicals.html

.

(11) University, Tulane, Online Learning, Community Sciences, Disaster Management, and Environmental Degrees. 2022. "The Role Of Public Health In Combating Environmental Toxins". Publichealth.Tul ane.Edu. https://publichealth.tulane.edu/blog/environmental-toxins/.

(12) "Fluorosis". 2022. Who.Int. https://www.who.int/teams/environment-climate-change-and-health/ water-sanitation-and-health/burden-of-disease/other-diseases-and-risks/fluorosis.

(13) Ducharme, Jamie. 2019. "Is Fluoride In Water Safe? A New Study Reignites That Long-Standing Debate". Time.
https://time.com/5656476/is-fluoride-in-water-safe/.
(14) Connett, Ph.D., Paul. 2012. "50 Reasons To Oppose Fluoridation". Fluoridealert.Org.
https://fluoridealert.org/articles/50-reasons/.
(15) Schmurak, Susannah. 2017. "Most Americans Drink Fluoridated Water. Is That A Good Thing?". Ensia.
https://ensia.com/features/fluoridated-water/.
(16) Consumer Reports. "4 Ways to Avoid PFAS in Your Water - Consumer Reports."
www.consumerreports.org, September 24, 2020.
https://www.consumerreports.org/water-quality/ways-to-avoid-pfas-in-your-water-a2126313336/.
(17) Consumer Reports. "What's Really in Your Bottled Water? - Consumer Reports."
www.consumerreports.org, September 24, 2020.
https://www.consumerreports.org/water-quality/whats-really-in-your-bottled-water-a5361150329/.
(18) Inan-Eroglu, Elif, and Aylin Ayaz. "Is Aluminum Exposure a Risk Factor for Neurological Disorders? - PMC."
National Institute of Health National Library of Medicine's National Center for Biotechnology Information.
www.ncbi.nlm.nih.gov, June 6, 2018.
https://www.ncbi.nlm.nih.gov/pmc/articles/PMC6040147/.
(19) SINC, Plataforma. "Espresso Makers: Coffee in Capsules Contains More Furan than the Rest."
ScienceDaily, April 14, 2011.
https://www.sciencedaily.com/releases/2011/04/110413090012.htm.
(20) https://www.compatible-capsules.com/category/coffee-sustainability/
(21) "2008 Biennial National Listing of Fish Advisories." EPA. Environmental Protection Agency.
https://www.epa.gov/guidance.
(22) US EPA, OAR. "Health Risk of Radon." Overviews and Factsheets, August 14, 2014.
https://www.epa.gov/radon/health-risk-radon.

(23) Foodnavigator.com. "Attention, algae! Food agency warns against carcinogenic contamination in edible seaweed." https://www.foodnavigator.com/Article/2020/08/27/Attention-algae!-Food-agency-warns-against-carcinogenic-contamination-in-edible-seaweed#.

(24) https://www.scientificamerican.com/article/ widely-used-herbicide-linked-to-cancer/

(25) https://www.epa.gov/indoor-air-quality-iaq/ does-epa-regulate-volatile-organic-compounds-vocs-household-products

(26) https://www.gardeningknowhow.com/ houseplants/hpgen/how-many-plants-for-clean-air-indoors.htm

(27) Cancer Treatment Centers of America. "What You Need to Know about Fasting and Cancer," June 9, 2021. https://www.cancercenter.com/community/blog/2021/06/fasting-cancer.

(28) MIT News / Massachusetts Institute of Technology. "Fasting Boosts Stem Cells' Regenerative Capacity." https://news.mit.edu/2018/fasting-boosts-stem-cells-regenerative-capacity-0503.

CHAPTER FOUR

GODDESSES EXERCISE

SUPERCHARGING YOUR LIFE

I regret that workout. ~ No one, ever

Goddesses must stay in training, because they never know when they'll be called on to save the world.

The Mayo Clinic says that too much sitting and prolonged periods of sitting increase the risk of death from cardiovascular disease and cancer. (29) Those who sit for eight hours a day with no physical activity have a risk of dying on par with that of smokers and obese individuals. Exercise can improve our balance, protect our bones, tighten and tone our body, help us maintain a healthy weight, expand our lung power, detoxify our bodies, strengthen our immune system, and protect against many age-related diseases. It can also improve our mental health, our outlook on life, and our memory! It's natural stress reduction. And get this, Goddess: We become biologically younger when we exercise! An older study by the National Institute of Health (2013) found that one minute of exercise increases lifespan by a full seven minutes. (30) That's an enviable return on investment.

Once women reach age 30 and beyond, a lack of exercise trumps smoking for increased risk of heart disease! Make sure you move your body every single day for at least 30-60 minutes. You can break this into several shorter sessions, such as two to four 15-minute walks. In fact, shorter, more frequent sessions are better for you because they help break up the time you spend being sedentary. I get busy researching and writing and can easily spend all day sitting unless I set a reminder to move every 60 minutes.

Exercise for the Goddess Brain

Researchers have found that exercise strengthens connections in our brain, particularly in the hippocampus. This is key because the hippocampus is the part of our brain responsible for memory, and it shrinks as we age, increasing our risk of memory loss and dementia. Regular exercise keeps the hippocampus strong.

Exercise also increases our ability to learn new things by accelerating brain cell production and forming new synaptic connections. We can rewire our brain with exercise!

Unfortunately, most of us don't get enough exercise, and many of us don't get the right kind of exercise. To maximize benefits, we should exercise to the point of sweating three to five times per week. And we should regularly get three types of exercise: aerobic (e.g., walking, swimming), strength (e.g., core exercises, weight training), and balance and flexibility (e.g., yoga, martial arts, stretching).

Rebounding

Rebounding is my go-to aerobic exercise. It involves exercising on a mini trampoline or rebounder. What's the difference between a mini-trampoline and a rebounder? About $300. I've used both and have found there's little difference between them.

Rebounding is gentle on the joints, yet it helps work muscles in the legs, increases endurance, and strengthens bones. Rebounding doesn't have to mean simply bouncing; that would bore me to death. The way I do it is easy, fun, and effective. I put on some great music and work out for six to eight songs (22-30 minutes). If I'm really feeling energetic, I'll go up to an hour. I alternate my movements with each song, jogging for one song, then high knees for the next. This keeps my workouts interesting and makes the time go by quickly. When I'm consistent with my rebounding, I like to push myself to go faster and faster. It's exhilarating. (I feel like Wonder Woman, but I've yet to reach hypersonic speed.)

Rebounding boosts balance and coordination and each time you catch air, your entire body pulls up, which supports the bladder, uterus, and bowel (pelvic floor).

Rebounding is the only exercise I know of that's both easy on the joints and helps improve the lymphatic and immune systems. The vertical bouncing, as opposed to the horizontal movements of running and other cardio, promotes the drainage and circulation of lymphatic fluids, draining toxins and other buildup and allowing our immune system to function optimally. Numerous articles reference a 1979 NASA study calling rebounding the "most efficient, effective exercise yet devised." (31) NASA selected rebounding as the best method to get astronauts back into shape after space travel deconditioning.

Need one more reason to rebound? Lymphatic drainage has great implications for displacement of cellulite. When the lymphatic system is functioning poorly, fat cells can swell, bunch up, and form that cottage cheese look we all love called cellulite. Regular rebounding can combat cellulite production and even reduce the cellulite we already have.

HIIT

Several years ago, I was complaining to a friend who is a fitness coach that I don't have time to work out. She asked, "What would you say if I told you that you could get a full workout in seven minutes?" I probably replied with something like, "That's crazy." But she knew something I didn't. She was talking about high-intensity interval training (HIIT). Not well known at the time, HIIT has become extremely popular for its ability to significantly increase physical fitness with short bursts of activity. HIIT involves repeated, short intervals of full-out exercise followed by periods of recovery at a moderate pace. This can be in the form of sprinting when you're out for a jog or increasing your pace on the treadmill or stationary bike to near-maximum capability for a brief time, then leveling off, then repeating. By forcing your body to switch between two vastly different states, you improve your cardio conditioning. This is more effective than keeping the same pace for a much longer time! And there's a bonus: It improves insulin sensitivity and blood pressure. You can even combine rebounding and HIIT; I've recommended one of my favorite combo workouts in your Goddess Gift for this chapter.

Strength Training

Strength training is one of the most important exercises we can do as we age. It increases bone density and strengthens connective tissues, preventing fractures and other injuries. It decreases body fat, builds muscle mass, and improves mental health. You don't even have to use weights! Simple strength training exercises that require no equipment include pushups, sit-ups, squats, planks, and Pilates.

Although you can strength train without any equipment, you may want to consider getting a bench press and bar bells or dumb bells. Strength training with a bench press opens up the ribs and chest, expanding the lungs, and this can reduce the risk of pneumonia.

Don't forget your core when strength training. Abdominal work, Pilates, and yoga all provide core strength training.

Aim for two strength training sessions per week.

Balance, Flexibility, and Crossing the Midline

Make certain you include some form of balance work in your exercise routine. Balance can diminish as we age, and poor balance is a cause of falls. Simply worrying about falling is also a cause of falls, so just do the exercises and forget about the worry! Some easy balance exercises are to stand with your weight on one leg, then raise the other leg to the side or behind you. Or cross the midline, bringing the leg you're not standing on out in front and to the side. Crossing the midline is important for mental health because it integrates both hemispheres of the brain.

Other balance exercises are found in yoga and Tai chi. Or walk heel to toe in a straight line as if you were pulled over for a sobriety test.

Strengthening our lower legs can also help with balance and prevent injuries. Toe raises and heel raises are great for this.

To increase flexibility, try stretching exercises, such as those found in yoga, or dynamic stretches, such as walking lunges, squats, or hula-hoop stretches (hands on hips, rotate your hips as if you were spinning a hula-hoop). Here's a great stretch for your chest, back, and arms that can even do seated: Bend your arms in front of you with your elbows at a 90-degree angle, hands in the air as if someone just said, "Stick 'em up!" Then, keeping the same 90-degree angle, move your arms and hands toward each other until they touch. Hold for a few seconds.

Lack Motivation? Great!

Motivation is an emotion, and just like any other emotion, it's transitory (nothing to hang your laurel wreath on)! Far more important than motivation is discipline. Discipline is true Goddess Power. With it, you do the work whether you feel motivated or not. Discipline is like a muscle. It may start off weak when you begin to use it, but every time you use it, it grows stronger. At first, it's hard! But after a while, you shift into autopilot. Exercise becomes something you just do, like brushing your teeth or feeding the cat. So, when you're not motivated to exercise, this is exactly the time to do it because it means you have the opportunity to strengthen your discipline superpower.

You don't have to belong to a gym to exercise. With the abundance of online workouts and exercise DVDs, and even the Home Mirror, with its subscription of in-home workouts, you can exercise in your home in any weather.

Exercise Tips

- Your weekly planner should include at least three vigorous aerobic workouts (or five moderate workouts), two strength workouts, and two balance and flexibility workouts.

- By switching up the types of exercise you do, you'll avoid boredom and work different muscle groups, increasing the benefits of exercise.
- Most people find it easier to stick to a routine if they schedule it first, before other distractions get in the way.
- Lay out workout clothes the night before. Have everything you need at the ready.
- Schedule a couple of workouts a week with a friend, someone you can count on.
- Get a dog for walking.
- Make it fun. Music, fun workout clothes, and walking to your favorite coffee shop are all ways to add enjoyment to your exercise routine.
- Set goals that get you excited, such as registering for a 5K or 10K walk or run.
- Create a chart with gold stars for each time you work out. After so many gold stars, reward yourself with a prize.
- Stand as often as possible. Create walk breaks instead of sitting all day. I keep an exercise chart by my desk that lists activities to do each hour: walk for two songs, 10 lunges, 10 pushups, 25 squats, etc.

Goddess Gift: Favorite Workouts

Following are some of my favorite online and offline workout videos:

- Fabulous 50s YouTube workouts on YouTube: cardio, strength, stretching, balance
- Leslie Sansone *Walk Away the Pounds* YouTube videos and DVDs
- POPSUGAR Fitness "Madonna Arms" YouTube video for toned arms
- *Yogalosophy* DVD, by Mandy Ingber for balance, strength, flexibility, and a total body workout
- HIIT/rebounder: "5 Minute Fat Burning Bellicon Interval Training Workout!" – YouTube video by Emily Chesher for aerobic conditioning and lymph draining

(29) Mayo Clinic. "Sitting Risks: How Harmful Is Too Much Sitting?"
https://www.mayoclinic.org/healthy-lifestyle/adult-health/
expert-answers/sitting/faq-20058005.
(30) "Every Minute of Exercise Could Lengthen Your Life Seven
Minutes."
https://www.wbur.org/news/2013/03/15/minutes-exercise-longer-life.
(31) MyFitnessPal Blog. "NASA, the Trampoline and You | Fitness |
MyFitnessPal," January 12, 2017.
https://blog.myfitnesspal.com/nasa-the-trampoline-and-you/.

CHAPTER FIVE

GODDESSES HYDRATE

OPTIMIZING LIQUID ENERGY

When the well is dry, we'll know the worth of water. ~ Benjamin Franklin

Did you know plants can feel gratitude? A few summers back, I was relaxing on my front porch, having just watered my parched shrubs and lawn. Overlooking the yard, I felt an outpouring of gratitude directed toward me. It was palpable. I could almost hear the plants saying, "Thank you for the water! We needed that!" The air, too, was charged with energy. It felt vibrant and alive. It was a feeling I'll never forget. You've probably witnessed a version of this yourself when a thirsty house plant "perked up" after receiving a dose of water.

Our bodies need water, too. Sometimes when I'm feeling tired or low, drinking a glass of water is all I need to give me a boost of energy. I feel renewed and refreshed. It's easy to get dehydrated without noticing it because our thirst signals are weak and are often disguised as hunger. By the time we realize we're thirsty, we're likely dehydrated. Dehydration is a health and psychological concern because it can impact our body's functions. It reduces our ability to control our temperature, reduces our motivation, and causes fatigue. The mere act of moving through life becomes more difficult, physically and mentally.

You may have heard that our bodies are two-thirds water, but did you know that our muscles have an even higher water content (80%)? Dehydration of as little as 1.4% of our body weight can leave us feeling lethargic, impair our mood and concentration, and can lead to headaches and constipation.

Water's Benefits

Staying hydrated improves mood and energy. It can also reduce our risk of kidney stones by increasing the amount of urine that passes through the kidneys, diluting the concentration of minerals, and making them less susceptible to forming stones. Water also helps our kidneys flush out toxins.

Water can even help us lose weight by boosting our metabolic rate and increasing the sensation of fullness—and it flushes out fat. Drinking water a half hour before meals may help us eat less. In a 2013 study of 50 overweight women, researchers found that drinking 16.9 oz (500 mL) of water before each meal for eight weeks led to significant reductions in body weight and body fat. (32) And drinking that same amount of water first thing in the morning can boost metabolism by 24%. (33)

Water is good for our skin, too. Dehydration makes our skin look dry and wrinkled, but water plumps it up, giving it a more youthful appearance. Skin contains lots of water and functions as a protective barrier to prevent excess fluid loss. For this purpose, healthful water is much better than expensive (often toxin-filled) moisturizing creams.

Water also carries nutrients and oxygen to our cells, flushes bacteria from our bladders, aids digestion, normalizes blood pressure, and stabilizes our heartbeat. It cushions joints, protects organs, tissues, and the spinal cord, and helps us maintain electrolyte (sodium) balance. But if you find getting eight glasses a day tough to swallow, there's good news.

How Much Water Is Enough?

It may not be necessary to drink eight glasses of water a day. Harvard Health researchers found that most people need about four to six cups of water each day, and that all beverages containing water contribute toward those daily needs—even coffee! (34) Their study found that while beverages containing caffeine or alcohol are dehydrating because they make us urinate, over the course of the day, the water from those beverages still contributes to a net positive in total fluid consumption. Water-rich foods such as celery, salads, and fruit also count. Water is always the best choice, but isn't it great to finally put that eight-glass requirement on ice?

Your needs for water will depend on your weight, the ambient temperature, your health, and your activity level. So, how can you be sure you're getting enough? Your body will tell you. If your urine is dark yellow, you're not getting enough. Clear? Probably plenty. And a lemon-yellow color is just right.

Healthy Water Reminder

As mentioned in the Goddesses Detox chapter, tap water may contain chemicals and toxins your body doesn't need. Getting a multi-step water filter is a good start. We already talked about avoiding plastic water bottles, but here's another reason to avoid them. Endocrine-disrupting chemicals can leach out of the plastic when the water bottles are exposed to heat (such as in a hot car, garage, shipping container, or warehouse). These can also leach out when the bottle is reused. The safest water bottles are those made from glass or stainless steel. Avoid aluminum bottles; these are often coated with chemicals, and aluminum is a toxin.

To Drink More Water

Here are some tips for adding more water to your life:

- Keep a toxic-free water bottle with you and refill it throughout the day.
- When dining out, opt for water over soda.
- Always serve water during meals.
- Add a slice of lemon, lime, or cucumber to your water.
- Add juice. I will often fill a glass one-quarter full of orange juice, then fill the rest with water. While juice isn't as healthy as plain water, limiting it to 25% of the glass helps me get more water in, and it's very tasty.
- Add mint leaves to your ice cube tray before filling it with water and freezing. Add these cubes to your water glass.
- Take a pinch of Himalayan salt (which contains more minerals than table salt) prior to drinking a glass of water. It can help your body absorb more water.
- Have beverages you enjoy! Mix up your water consumption with plain coffee or tea, sparkling water, seltzers, and flavored waters (avoiding sugar and artificial ingredients).
- Avoid sports drinks, which are often flavored with chemicals.
- Eat more fruits and vegetables. The higher water content is just one of the many benefits of these power foods. Fruits and veggies such as spinach, watermelon, cantaloupe, tomatoes, kiwi, cabbage, celery, pickles, oranges, and squash are made up of 90-99% water. (Don't look to corn, peas, or potatoes for water content; these are not nearly as hydrating.)
- Soup is also a great option for hydration if you opt for clear or vegetable-based soups. Gazpacho, often called a "liquid salad," is a delicious choice.
- Prior to exercising, drink two glasses of water, and sip water frequently during workout sessions to replace fluids lost through sweat.
- Place a checkmark on your calendar for each glass of water you drink each day. This will help you keep track and ensure you're getting enough. Or fill a container with a day's worth of water and drink from it throughout the day.

Reverse Osmosis Water

Perhaps you've heard of reverse osmosis water treatment systems and wondered what the buzz is about. Although it's meant to be healthier, stripping out toxins and delivering a fresh taste, low-mineral drinking water produced by reverse osmosis or distillation isn't suitable for long-term human consumption according to the WHO. A high-quality activated carbon filter (the Berkey system mentioned earlier, for example) is more convenient, less wasteful, less expensive, and retains healthy minerals in the water.

Alkaline Water

You'll sometimes see bottled water sold as alkaline water. Proponents say it can neutralize acid in the bloodstream. However, research shows that it's unlikely to significantly impact pH levels in blood. When you drink alkaline water, you merely change the pH of what's in your toilet bowl, not what's in your blood. When the alkaline water hits your stomach, the acids in your gut neutralize it. So, you'll end up paying more money to drink something that won't lower your body's acidity. According to the Mayo Clinic, there's little evidence that drinking alkaline water prevents diseases, such as cancer or heart disease, despite reports otherwise. (35) Short-term use may help prevent some bone loss, but the evidence isn't clear.

Supercharging Your Water

Want to bring water to the next level? Substitute one to two glasses of water a day with these supercharged water options.

Lemon Water

Squeezing a bit of lemon juice into your water can promote weight loss. The polyphenol antioxidants found in lemons were found to reduce weight gain significantly in mice that were overfed to induce obesity. It also helped to improve insulin resistance and lowered other markers that can lead to type 2 diabetes.

Lemon water can also improve skin quality. The vitamin C in lemons helps reduce skin wrinkling, dry skin, and sun damage.

Lemon water also aids digestion, and a cup of warm lemon water in the morning can help wake up the digestive system. Make it part of your morning routine to help prevent constipation.

Diatomaceous Earth

Taking food-grade diatomaceous earth is safe and healthy. It can help detox heavy metals in the body and kill pathogens. Make sure you get the food grade, non-crystallized form, not the kind used as a pest control.

Diatomaceous earth (DE) is cool stuff! It's made of prehistoric fossilized phytoplankton. This phytoplankton consumes silica and when the plankton dies, it leaves the shell at the bottom of the seabed. The benefit is in the silica, which is the second most prevalent element on the planet. Silica is great for strong nails and healthy hair, and it gives skin a fuller, less wrinkly look. Silica is also good for tendons and supports the aorta and the health of bones and teeth. I find that my joints feel smoother since I've started adding DE to my daily routine.

Take one teaspoon a day on an empty stomach (it has very little taste, simply a mild chalky flavor that's not unpleasant). Simply pour a small glass of water, add a teaspoon of diatomaceous earth, stir well, and drink all at once. If a bit of residue remains in your glass, add more water, stir, and drink.

Apple Cider Vinegar

Adding a tablespoon of apple cider vinegar (ACV) to an 8-ounce glass of water is an easy way to improve your body's alkalinity. ACV includes antimicrobial and antioxidant properties, and evidence suggests it may have other health benefits, such as aiding weight loss, reducing cholesterol, and lowering blood sugar levels, which can improve symptoms of diabetes. Look for apple cider vinegar with a label that reads "with the mother." This unfiltered and unrefined vinegar has a cloudy and murky appearance due to the presence of beneficial bacteria, yeast, and protein. The healing properties of ACV are due to the presence of acetic acid and other beneficial compounds. These are removed when the vinegar is processed into the clear, non-mother version.

Goddess Gift: Water Facts

- Water regulates the Earth's temperature and your temperature as well.
- Nearly 97% of the Earth's water is salty or otherwise undrinkable.
- There is the same amount of water on Earth as there was when the Earth was formed. This means that water from your tap could contain molecules that dinosaurs drank!
- The human brain is 75% water, just like trees.
- Tears carry natural pain killers, flush out stress hormones and toxins, and release oxytocin and endorphins, helping to ease both physical and emotional pain. The type of tears formed from emotional pain contain more of these pain killers than those caused by an eye irritant. Go ahead, have a good cry! It's good for you.

(32) Davy, Brenda M., Elizabeth A. Dennis, A. Laura Dengo, Kelly L. Wilson, and Kevin P. Davy. "Water Consumption Reduces Energy Intake at a Breakfast Meal in Obese Older Adults." Journal of the American Dietetic Association 108, no. 7 (July 2008): 1236–39. https://doi.org/10.1016/j.jada.2008.04.013.

(33) Dubnov-Raz, G., N. W. Constantini, H. Yariv, S. Nice, and N. Shapira. "Influence of Water Drinking on Resting Energy Expenditure in Overweight Children." International Journal of Obesity (2005) 35, no. 10 (October 2011): 1295–1300. https://doi.org/10.1038/ijo.2011.130.

(34) Harvard Health. "How Much Water Should You Drink?," September 6, 2016. https://www.health.harvard.edu/staying-healthy/how-much-water-should-you-drink.

(35) Mayo Clinic. "Alkaline Water: Better than Plain Water?"
https://www.mayoclinic.org/healthy-lifestyle/
nutrition-and-healthy-eating/expert-answers/
alkaline-water/faq-20058029.

CHAPTER SIX

GODDESS HEALTHCARE

CHAMPIONING YOUR HEALTH

The art of medicine consists of amusing the patient while nature cures the disease. ~ Voltaire

Your Goddess body is wise and beautiful. Pharmaceuticals have their place but are often abused and overprescribed, to deleterious effect. We've only begun to realize the impact of overprescribing antibiotics: Antibiotic-resistant infection treatment costs have doubled since 2002 and in 2018 were more than $2.2 billion annually. (36) Worse is the loss of human life. The Centers for Disease Control and Prevention (CDC) estimates that 23,000 Americans die due to antibiotic resistant infections each year. (37)

One reason medications are often overprescribed is the incentive for doing so. Kickbacks are illegal, but pharmaceutical companies can pay doctors in other ways for promoting their products: public speaking fees, consulting fees, meals, and travel. Drug company perks and rewards have been found to increase doctor recommendations for prescriptions. In one study by Cornell University, it was found that for every dollar drug companies spent on marketing to doctor's offices, they could expect to receive $2.64 in revenue, a 164% return on investment. (38) Want to know if your doctor is receiving funds from Big Pharma? Check at openpaymentsdata.cms.gov.

Medication: Too Much of a Good Thing?

At age 50-something I visited my doctor for an annual checkup. I'm sure I passed through the Precambrian, Paleozoic, Mesozoic, and Cenozoic Eras before I was finally ushered to an exam room. The physician's assistant reviewed my chart on a screen, then looked at me, eyes wide. "I've never seen anyone your age who wasn't on some kind of medication."

That surprised me. I wasn't that old, I thought. But I likely was that naïve. According to the Georgetown University Health Policy Institute, chronic illness has most older adults on prescription drugs, including 75% of those age 50 to 64. This jumps to 91% at age 80. And the average number of prescriptions used also increases with age: from 13 for those age 50 to 64 to 22 for those age 80 and older. (39)

Polypharmacy is the term for taking multiple medications simultaneously. All drugs have side effects, and drug interactions are risky because it's difficult to calibrate medications appropriately when combined. According to agingcare.com, "Polypharmacy in the elderly is a major contributor to disability, frailty, falls, long-term care placement, and a decreased quality of life." (40) Negative symptoms of polypharmacy are often attributed to aging rather than what they are—overmedication. Common adverse symptoms from polypharmacy include confusion, sleepiness, loss of appetite, digestion issues, falls and other mobility issues, depression, weakness, tremors, hallucinations, anxiety, dizziness, changes in sexual behavior, and skin rashes.

To prevent issues related to polypharmacy, stay as healthy as you can so that medications aren't needed in the first place. Keep a list of all prescription medications and their dosage, and keep this list updated. Read package inserts for contraindications. If you can't locate the package insert, you can look it up on the DailyMed database of the National Library of Medicine:

dailymed.nlm.nih.gov/dailymed/index.cfm

It's also helpful to use the same pharmacy for all medications because your pharmacist can be another line of defense against polypharmacy errors.

Prescription Medicines

A study in England found that one-tenth of items dispensed by primary care physicians were inappropriately prescribed. (41) The more prescription medications taken, the higher the chance that one or more of them will have harmful effects. For any prescription medication you take, discuss with your doctor whether there is a plan for tapering off. All medications have side effects, and there may be healthier alternatives you can explore while gradually weaning yourself from the medication. If a medication is something your doctor says you must take for the rest of your life, get a second opinion, research, and consider consulting a naturopath.

Before taking a new medication, make certain your doctor is aware of any allergies you have and any other prescription medications you're taking. Mention any natural supplements, herbs, vitamins, or over-the-counter meds you're on as well. Some may conflict with that new prescription you're about to fill, either by reducing its efficacy or by causing unwanted side effects. Some foods conflict with medications as well, so check with your healthcare provider.

Two prescription medications deserve special attention here. As much as possible, avoid **steroids** in any form. These reduce, even eliminate, stem cell viability. **Antibiotics** are also problematic. The CDC says that one in three antibiotic prescriptions is unnecessary, with amoxicillin being the most common. (42) Overuse of antibiotics can destroy gut flora and can lead to antibiotic-resistance. If you must take an antibiotic, ask your doctor how to supplement with a probiotic without reducing the antibiotic's efficacy. Protecting your gut during a round of antibiotics can keep you from ending up with a yeast infection, urinary tract infection, or C. difficile. A healthy gut helps fight cancer and aids in digestion, weight maintenance, and overall good health.

An over-the-counter medication often prescribed by doctors is **Tylenol**. While it's been around for years, and most of us have a bottle of it in our medicine cabinets, it carries risk. Just one quadruple dose can cause death. Due to intense lobbying by its manufacturer, the FDA has been slow to improve warnings on the over-the-counter version of Tylenol, but it has required wording regarding the potential for liver damage to labels. (43) Acetaminophen has also been linked to asthma and is therefore contraindicated for those with a respiratory infection. If you've been prescribed Tylenol in any form, ask your doctor about risks and alternatives.

Discuss any medication you're on with your doctor at least annually (and certainly any time you experience an adverse effect). Ask why the medication is necessary. Can it be discontinued, or its dosage reduced? Is there a safer substitute?

Are You Over-Screening?

Medical screenings carry both risks and benefits and should be considered carefully in consultation with your medical provider. In contrast to diagnostic testing, screenings are performed on healthy individuals who show no symptoms of disease. And according to a report at cancer.gov, many older adults are over-screened. (44) At some point, we "age out" of the need for cancer screening because the risk associated with the screening is greater than the potential reward from being screened. While the U.S. Preventative Services Task Force (USPSTF) recommends that all adults get screened for colon cancer from age 50 every 10 years until at least age 75, a study performed by University of Texas researchers found that nearly a quarter of colonoscopies performed on Texas Medicare patients aged 70 and older were inappropriate due to the patients' age and estimated risks for colon cancer. (45) So, in addition to risk factors, we should consider life expectancy and overall health. A healthy 80-year-old may opt for screenings that a 65-year-old with end-stage Alzheimer's disease may choose to avoid. And if the answer is no to the following question, the screening is likely unnecessary: "If we were to find something, would you take any action?"

Mammograms

For women in the U.S. with no cancer history, screening guidelines for routine mammograms ends at age 75. And while annual mammogram screening is recommended for women aged 45-54, switching to every two years is routinely recommended for women aged 55 and older. However, a UW-Madison study found that most women aged 50-74 should consider getting mammograms every three years instead of every two to reduce the risks associated with breast cancer screening. (46) Mammograms expose breasts to low-level radiation and often convey false positives that require further testing, such as biopsies, which carry their own risks. The Mayo Clinic recommends that all women take the following measures to reduce their risk of breast cancer: limit alcohol to no more than one drink per day, maintain a healthy weight, be physically active, breast-feed (the benefits increase the longer you breast-feed), and limit postmenopausal hormone therapy. (47)

Past a certain age, mammograms may not be medically necessary. An abstract in the *Journal of General Internal Medicine* (April 2022), states that while guidelines recommend against routine screening for breast, colorectal, and prostate cancer in older adults with less than 10 years of life expectancy, physicians often continue to recommend screening for these patients. (48)

You have the right to refuse any screening. You also have a right to request screening if you're healthy and have a concern that screening will alleviate. You may need to make a case for medical necessity to get it covered by your insurance carrier, however.

Beyond Allopathic Medicine

Conventional (allopathic or mainstream) medicine, the most well-known type of healthcare in most western countries, consists of a primary doctor, specialists, and nursing staff providing care through medication, surgery, radiation, and other therapies and procedures. Its popularity is due in no small part to the fact that it's the form of healthcare most likely to be covered by insurance providers. However, it's by no means the only option.

Osteopathy care doctors are licensed physicians and surgeons in the U.S. and carry the title DO instead of MD. Some areas outside the U.S. don't recognize osteopaths, but they undergo the same residency requirements as other doctors. DOs are more likely to recommend complementary treatments outside of mainstream medicine than are their MD counterparts.

Complementary and **integrative** medicine are healthcare options that can be used along with mainstream medicine. These may include holistic medicine, homeopathy, functional medicine, naturopathy, chiropractic care, Chinese medicine, and Ayurveda. Often called "alternative" medicine, these types of healthcare meet the definition of alternative only when used in lieu of, not in addition to, allopathic care.

Holistic medicine is a layered approach to healthcare used with other modalities. The holistic practitioner employs a whole body, mind, spirit, and emotional approach to health and wellness.

Homeopathy uses an approach of minimal dosage and "like curing like" with the belief that a lower dose of medication has a greater effect than a higher dose due to the way the body responds. Homeopaths often treat illness and disease with herbs that would cause a similar response in healthy people. These may include arnica or belladonna for pain, or marigold (Calendula) for wound care.

Functional medicine is a holistic, biology-based approach to health that looks to food and fasting as medicine. It focuses on lifestyle modifications, including nutrition and helps clients avoid highly inflammatory foods such as gluten, dairy, corn, peanuts, artificial sweeteners, and sugar. Functional medicine is said to focus on the "person who has the disease" rather than the "disease the person has" and uses genetics, lifestyle, and environment to diagnose and treat dysfunction and imbalance.

Naturopaths are trained as primary care providers and can diagnose, prevent, and treat illness. Like other non-allopathic practitioners, rather than focusing on symptoms, naturopaths look for the underlying cause of a disease or illness and then apply nature-based treatments to work in concert with the natural healing mechanisms of the body.

Chinese medicine focuses on balancing a person's life force, called qi (pronounced "chee"). Yin and yang are the opposite and complementary forces that make up our qi. Treatments employed by Chinese medicine practitioners include acupuncture, cupping, massage, herbal remedies, and movement exercises, such as tai chi. I've had little experience with Chinese medicine, but once, when nothing else had worked, I went to an acupuncturist for a neck injury. Barely able to move my head, I was placed on a table and multiple needles were inserted into my forehead, knees, and wrists. Then the practitioner left me alone in a dark room for 45 minutes. Thanks a lot. Finally, the practitioner came in and removed the needles. I was thinking, "What a crock" as I went to pay for my visit at the front desk and couldn't wait to answer the question, "How do you feel?" with a complaint. Then I realized I had absolutely no pain or stiffness in my neck and had regained full mobility. Silly grasshopper.

Chiropractic care focuses on the spine and body joints and their connections to the nervous system. Chiropractors make adjustments to restore mobility. I've had great chiropractors and horrible chiropractors, so I recommend getting a referral from someone you trust. Once, though, I didn't have time for a referral and ended up going to a chiropractic clinic that specialized in sports medicine. I had tweaked my back so badly that I was in excruciating pain. I walked to the front door like Tim Conway's old man in *The Carol Burnett Show* and stood while waiting to be seen because I could not sit down. When the chiropractor brought me back to the examining room, he eased me onto a padded metal table, rolled my back with a heated "iron," and dropped parts of my body several times using levers on the table. By the time I left I was 50% better. We scheduled a second appointment a few days later, after which I was 80% better, and by the end of the third appointment, I was fine. Almost a year to the day, I did something similar to my back and returned to the clinic with similar results. Chiropractic medicine has its place, and I'm grateful for it.

Ayurveda is self-care medicine that's more than 5,000 years old; it's one of India's traditional health care modalities. Ayurveda relies on plant, animal, metal, and mineral products and extracts plus diet, exercise, and lifestyle choices. Like Chinese medicine, it focuses on energy balance, but in this case, it is the balance among three life forces (doshas): Vata dosha (space and air); Pitta dosha (fire and water); and Kapha dosha (water and earth). According to the National Center for Complementary and Integrative Health, conventional and Ayurvedic treatments for rheumatoid arthritis were found to be similarly effective, with the conventional drug methotrexate compared to the Ayurvedic treatment, which involved 40 herbal compounds. (49) In another study, 500 mg of curcumin (found in turmeric) was found to be more effective in pain reduction than 50 mg of diclofenac sodium, an anti-inflammatory drug. (50) Like any medical treatment, Ayurveda used haphazardly without the guidance of a skilled practitioner (for instance, ingesting tinctures purchased online that claim to be Ayurvedic is unwise). I have limited experience with Ayurveda medicine, but I am impressed by its 5,000-year history and intend to learn more about it.

My three primary healthcare providers are me, myself, and I. I believe that we each know our own bodies best and when we choose a healthy lifestyle that includes exercise, eating right, reducing stress, reducing toxins, maintaining healthy connections, mindfulness, hydration, and appropriate sleep, we are our own best doctor. Depending on what I need, I may see a naturopath, an acupuncturist, a chiropractor, or an integrative medicine doctor. It has been nearly 10 years since that physician's assistant said, "I've never seen anyone your age who wasn't on some kind of medication," and I'm still not.

Goddess Gift: Home Remedies

Turmeric-Ginger Tea

Because inflammation is at the root of most illness and disease, reducing inflammation is a great preventive measure you can take. Curcumin (found in turmeric) is prized for its anti-inflammation properties, but it's hard to ingest enough natural turmeric to see a therapeutic benefit. Curcumin supplements may be one answer. If you prefer the root turmeric, consider this delicious "tea." Grate turmeric and ginger roots into a teapot. Add freshly ground black pepper (which boosts curcumin's benefits by as much as 2,000%). Pour in boiling water and allow it to steep covered for eight minutes. Add lemon juice and honey if desired.

Muscle Pain Relief

Did you know that chili peppers have been used for pain management? Capsaicin is the active ingredient. Create your own healthy salve for sore muscles by adding 3 tablespoons of cayenne powder to 1 cup of coconut oil in a saucepan. Heat over low heat, stirring occasionally, until the oil melts. Pour it into a bowl, allow it to become firm, and use as a balm when it's cooled. Avoid using this around your face or eyes.

Beef Up Your Bone Broth

Shitake mushrooms contain lentinan, which promotes antioxidant and anti-inflammatory effects. Studies have shown that it can inhibit breast cancer cells and may help fight other types of cancer. Try adding a few shitake mushrooms to your bone broth.

Buttermilk: "Out, Damned (Age) Spot!"

Buttermilk contains both lactic and ascorbic acid. Studies have shown that the combination of these two can lighten age spots more than lactic acid alone. Apply with a swab or cotton ball and rinse with water after 20 minutes.

Do you know of some great healthy home remedies? I'd love to hear about them! Write me at yvonneaileen@gmail.com.

(36) Thorpe, Kenneth E., Peter Joski, and Kenton J. Johnston. "Antibiotic-Resistant Infection Treatment Costs Have Doubled Since 2002, Now Exceeding $2 Billion Annually." Health Affairs 37, no. 4 (April 1, 2018): 662–69.
https://doi.org/10.1377/hlthaff.2017.1153.
(37) CDC. "The Biggest
Antibiotic-Resistant Threats in the U.S." Centers for Disease Control and Prevention, March 29, 2022.
https://www.cdc.gov/drugresistance/biggest-threats.html.
(38) WebMD. "Drug Company Perks Spur Doctors' Prescriptions."
https://www.webmd.com/drug-medication/news/20200221/
brand-name-rx-rise-after-docs-get-drug-company-perks-study.

(39) Health Policy Institute. "Prescription Drugs." Accessed April 17, 2022.

https://hpi.georgetown.edu/rxdrugs/.

(40) "Polypharmacy in the Elderly: Taking Too Many Medications Can Be Risky."

https://www.agingcare.com/articles/ polypharmacy-dangerous-drug-interactions-119947.htm.

(41) Mahase, Elisabeth. "Overprescribing: 10% of Items Dispensed in Primary Care Are Inappropriate, Review Finds." BMJ 374 (September 22, 2021): n2338.

https://doi.org/10.1136/bmj.n2338.

(42) CDC. "CDC Newsroom," January 1, 2016.

https://www.cdc.gov/media/releases/2016/ p0503-unnecessary-prescriptions.html.

(43) Miller, Jeff Gerth and T. Christian. "Tylenol Can Kill You." Business Insider.

https://www.businessinsider.com/tylenol-can-kill-you-2013-9.

(44) "Older Adults Often Unnecessarily Screened for Cancer - National Cancer Institute." CgvBlogPost, August 27, 2020.

https://www.cancer.gov/news-events/cancer-currents-blog/ 2020/screening-cancer-older-adults-unnecessary.

(45) Sheffield, Kristin M., Yimei Han, Yong-Fang Kuo, Taylor S. Riall, and James S. Goodwin. "Potentially Inappropriate Screening Colonoscopy in Medicare Patients: Variation by Physician and Geographic Region." JAMA Internal Medicine 173, no. 7 (April 8, 2013): 542–50.

https://doi.org/10.1001/jamainternmed.2013.2912.

(46) Newspapers, DAVID WAHLBERG Lee. "Many Women Could Get Mammograms Every Three Years, UW Study Says." Journal Times. Accessed April 17, 2022.

https://journaltimes.com/many-women-could-get-mammograms- every-three-years-uw-study-says/article_6bc0d686-40c2-5801-9413- 1c1c11609b73.html.

(47) Mayo Clinic. "Breast Cancer - Symptoms and Causes."

https://www.mayoclinic.org/diseases-conditions/ breast-cancer/symptoms-causes/syc-20352470.

(48) Enns, Justine P., Craig E. Pollack, Cynthia M. Boyd, Jacqueline Massare, and Nancy L. Schoenborn. "Discontinuing Cancer Screening for Older Adults: A Comparison of Clinician Decision-Making for Breast, Colorectal, and Prostate Cancer Screenings." Journal of General Internal Medicine 37, no. 5 (April 2022): 1122–28.
https://doi.org/10.1007/s11606-021-07121-9.

(49) NCCIH. "Ayurvedic Medicine: In Depth." Accessed April 17, 2022. https://www.nccih.nih.gov/health/ayurvedic-medicine-in-depth.

(50) Shep, Dhaneshwar, Chitra Khanwelkar, Prakashchandra Gade, and Satyanand Karad. "Safety and Efficacy of Curcumin versus Diclofenac in Knee Osteoarthritis: A Randomized Open-Label Parallel-Arm Study." Trials 20, no. 1 (April 11, 2019): 214.
https://doi.org/10.1186/s13063-019-3327-2.

CHAPTER SEVEN

GODDESS BRAIN POWER

STAYING GODDESS SHARP FOR LIFE

Dementia is not a normal part of aging. ~ National Institute on Aging, U.S. Department of Health & Human Services

One reason people fear aging is the belief that with it unavoidably comes senility, dementia, and memory loss. It can, but it doesn't have to. Alzheimer's disease is the most common form of dementia, and it affects more than 6 million Americans. In reality, it affects many other: the unpaid caregivers of those individuals: often spouses, adult children, or other loved ones. Alzheimer's disease kills more people than breast cancer and prostate cancer combined. Novelist Nicholas Sparks (*The Notebook*) calls it "a thief of hearts and souls and memories."

However, Alzheimer's disease is not the boogie man, lurking in the shadows, waiting to pounce. It's merely a disease of the brain, just as coronary artery disease is a disease of the heart. As with other afflictions of aging, you can reduce your risk of contracting it through healthy lifestyle choices. According to Harvard Health, in only 1% of cases genes determine whether you will have Alzheimer's. (51) These three genes relate to amyloid-beta production. For the other 99% of cases, the causes are multifaceted and may include inflammation in the brain, vascular factors, impacts of lifestyle choices. And even for that 1% there's hope. Genetic makeup is fixed, but the expression of those genes is not. An entire field of science—epigenetics—is based on the understanding that we can modify the expression of our genes.

The National Health Service (NHS) in England recommends you reduce your risk of cardiovascular disease, because this has been linked to both Alzheimer's and vascular dementia, caused by reduced blood flow to the brain. Per the NHS, to reduce the risk of these conditions and also prevent strokes and heart attacks, adhere to the following healthy lifestyle choices. (52)

- Don't smoke.
- Drink alcohol only in moderation, if at all.
- Eat a healthy, balanced diet, including at least five servings of fruit and vegetables each day and limit sugar.

> The Mediterranean diet is an excellent choice because it includes fresh vegetables and fruits, whole grains, olive oil, nuts, legumes, fish, moderate amounts of poultry, eggs, and dairy, and moderate amounts of red wine, with red meat consumed only rarely. A high fat diet plus copper-containing foods (organ meats, peanuts, legumes) increases your risk of Alzheimer's. Omega-3 DHA helps protect the brain against cell damage that can cause Alzheimer's, while leafy greens, carrots, turmeric (curcumin) can suppress amyloid production (reducing amyloid plaques, which play a role in Alzheimer's disease).

- Get moderate-intensity cardio exercise at least three to four days each week. Exercise stimulates blood flow to your brain and reduces your risk for high blood pressure, which has been associated with dementia.
- Control your blood pressure.

- Maintain a healthy weight and avoid type 2 diabetes. (Type 2 diabetes is so strongly correlated to Alzheimer's disease that Alzheimer's is often referred to as type 3 diabetes.)
- Stay mentally and socially active: reading, learning foreign languages, playing musical instruments, volunteering in your community, participating in group sports such as bowling, trying new activities or hobbies, and maintaining an active social life. A study in *Neurology* found that regular reading and writing late in life reduced the rate of memory decline by 32%. (53) And exercise increases neuroplasticity.
- Get enough sleep. Harvard Health reports that improved sleep can help prevent Alzheimer's disease and is linked to greater amyloid clearance from the brain. Aim for seven to eight hours each night. (54)

Other Tips

Strive for good posture. Maintaining an upright posture improves circulation and blood flow to the brain. Avoid risk factors for Alzheimer's, such as hearing loss, untreated depression, loneliness or social isolation, and a sedentary lifestyle. And consider intermittent fasting. Research on its potential benefits for the prevention of dementia is still in preliminary stages, but it has been shown to be a promising approach to preventing vascular dementia. A report by the U.S. National Library of Medicine at the National Institutes of Health found an association between vascular dementia and dietary patterns, "... Suggesting that dietary regulation leads to better control of energy metabolism, improvements in brain insulin resistance, and the suppression of neuroinflammation." (55) Benefits were found in the areas of neuroinflammation, synaptic plasticity, vascular function, insulin resistance, and neurogenesis. The article concluded, "We suggest that the application of intermittent fasting may be an effective dietary therapy for preventing the onset and/or suppressing the development of dementia."

An easy start to intermittent fasting is to limit your feeding window to 12 hours per day. For instance, have your last meal end at 7 p.m.

and don't eat again until 7 a.m. Because most of this time will be spent sleeping, this is doable for most of us. A 16/8 fasting-to-feeding window might have you delaying breakfast until 11 a.m.

At any given age, our brains are better at some activities than others. MIT researchers in cognitive science found that our brain processing power and detail memory peaks at age 18, the ability to learn unfamiliar names at age 22, facial recognition at age 32, concentration at age 43, the ability to learn and understand new information at age 50, and our vocabulary skills at age 67. (56) Take that, Tik Toker! The world doesn't fully belong to the young!

When we age, our brain shrinks and the blood flow within the brain slows. The brain loses volume, causing a loss of some nerve cell connections. Memory lapses occur more often. This is not dementia, but it can be disconcerting. To prevent this, exercise your brain by learning new skills, working on crossword puzzles, and staying active and social. Remain curious and be a lifelong learner. Take classes. Take up new hobbies. And make sure you're getting a good balance of omega-3 fatty acids (from supplementation or wild salmon and other wild fish, for instance).

Brain Nutrition

Foods that have been linked to better brain power are leafy greens (kale, spinach, collards, broccoli), fatty fish, such as salmon (wild caught), blueberries (aim for two or more servings each week), tea and coffee (for the caffeine, which has been linked to better mental function and storing new memories), walnuts (linked to improved memory), turmeric (for curcumin, which can cross the blood-brain barrier and is associated with reduced inflammation), pumpkin seeds (high in several micronutrients important to brain health), dark chocolate (70% or greater cocoa content), foods rich in vitamin C (oranges, bell peppers, guava, kiwi, tomatoes), eggs (for choline, used to create acetylcholine, a neurotransmitter that helps regulate mood and memory), and green tea (for its polyphenols and antioxidants, which can protect the brain from mental decline, reduce the risk of Alzheimer's and Parkinson diseases, and may also be associated with improved memory function.

The Mayo Clinic recommends the MIND diet for brain health, which is a blend of the DASH diet (Dietary Approaches to Stop Hypertension) and the Mediterranean diet. The MIND diet consists of leafy greens (at least six servings of leafy greens a week), two or more servings of berries per week, a handful of nuts at least five times a week (aim for a half-cup to a full cup of beans, nuts, and seeds per day), and olive oil instead of other seed oils. You should not heat olive oil because its health benefits (antioxidants and phenolic compounds) are degraded by heating. Instead, use MCT oil, coconut oil, or avocado oil for cooking. For protein, the MIND diet recommends consuming red meat no more than four times per week and choosing beans or lentils as alternate protein sources. Fish should be eaten once per week (again, wild-caught, not farmed) and limit alcohol to one serving daily. Alcohol can increase blood flow, making it less susceptible to clotting but consume it in moderation.

Goddess Gift: Brain Foods

Try to incorporate these ingredients into your favorite recipes (as alternatives to less healthy options) for their brain-boosting power:

Avocados: 60% of the brain is made up of fat and half of that is from omega-3s. Avocados are an excellent source of omega-3.

Walnuts are shaped like a brain for a reason! They've been shown to help lower blood pressure and improve brain function.

Dark chocolate: Cacao has high doses of antioxidants plus the plant compound flavanol, which has anti-inflammatory effects. It has also been shown to reduce blood pressure and get more blood flow to your brain.

Blueberries are linked to slower mental decline.

(51) *Harvard Health. "What Can You Do to Avoid Alzheimer's Disease?,"* January 13, 2017.
https://www.health.harvard.edu/alzheimers-and-dementia/ what-can-you-do-to-avoid-alzheimers-disease.

(52) National Institutes of Health (NIH). "Combination of Healthy Lifestyle Traits May Substantially Reduce Alzheimer's," June 17, 2020.
https://www.nih.gov/news-events/news-releases/combination-healthy-lifestyle-traits-may-substantially-reduce-alzheimers.

(53) Melnyk, Rebecca. "Memory Declines Much Slower in People Who Read, Write throughout Life: U.S. Study." National Post, July 4, 2013.
https://nationalpost.com/health/memory-declines-much-slower-in-peop who-read-write-throughout-life-u-s-study.

(54) Harvard Health. "What Can You Do to Avoid Alzheimer's Disease?," January 13, 2017.
https://www.health.harvard.edu/alzheimers-and-dementia/ what-can-you-do-to-avoid-alzheimers-disease.

(55) Yoon, Gwangho, and Juhyun Song. "Intermittent Fasting: A Promising Approach for Preventing Vascular Dementia." Journal of Lipid and Atherosclerosis 8, no. 1 (May 2019):
1–7. https://doi.org/10.12997/jla.2019.8.1.1.

(56) Griffiths, Josie, and The Sun. "This the Exact Age When Your Brain Power Peaks." New York Post (blog), August 1, 2017.
https://nypost.com/2017/08/01/ this-the-exact-age-when-your-brain-power-peaks/.

CHAPTER EIGHT

GODDESS MINDFULNESS AND MINDSET

AWAKENING YOUR SUPERPOWERS

You should sit in meditation for twenty minutes every day—unless you're too busy; then you should sit for an hour.
~ Dr. Sukhraj Dhillon

Mindset

Mindset is our fixed attitude toward life, one that can predetermine our response to or interpretation of an event or situation. Is that glass half full or half empty? Our mindset is the lens through which we perceive the world. What we think matters, quite literally. Quantum physics tells us that thoughts create vibrations in the energy field that surrounds us, and these can impact the material world. Imagine that! Albert Einstein, in his famous $e=mc^2$ demonstrated how energy and matter are connected. Scientists have discovered that matter and energy are not only connected, but also one and the same. This is known as particle-wave duality. Inside the smallest bit of matter is energy in motion. The atom is not matter but "empty space." So is the air we breathe, our bodies, and our tissues. But because this empty space is dense energy in constant motion, it appears as solid matter. Do some googling on the "observer effect" and the "entanglement theory" of quantum mechanics and prepare to have your mind blown.

As the placebo effect demonstrates, we're not only what we eat, but we're also what we think. Our inner dialogue, positive or negative, can impact our health at the cellular level. Countless studies demonstrate that just thinking about something can cause the brain to emit neurotransmitters—chemical messengers that allow it to communicate with itself and our nervous system. Neurotransmitters control nearly all of our body's functions, from hormone regulation to digestion to mood and stress level. In this way, and so many more, a thought is a tangible thing that influences other tangible things.

Negative thoughts result in chemical reactions that increase bodily stress and decrease immune function. Negative thinking comes in many forms. It may involve blaming yourself, focusing only on the negative aspects of an event or situation, or nuclear thinking (imagining the worst possible outcome for a given situation). Often, we're unaware that we've become a "glass half empty" person. Ask yourself how you would complete the following sentences. Try to come up with two to three responses for each sentence:

I am ...
My health is ...
My ability to earn income is ...
My wealth is ...
People find me ...
In social situations, I ...
My love life is ...
My ability to attract positive outcomes is ...

Negative thoughts have negative outcomes. So, if you find yourself having a negative thought, such as "I'll never fix this problem," or "I'll never be able to afford that trip," stop and shift your inner dialogue to "Every day I take steps to achieve optimum health" and "I'm always able to afford everything I need." Beyond merely feeling good and the health benefits, positive self-talk can translate into positive outcomes in the real world because they allow the creative space to make the positive thoughts come to fruition.

Take Advantage of Cognitive Dissonance

Cognitive dissonance is a psychological term that means we're uncomfortable holding two conflicting beliefs or thoughts. So, if you believe you can't do something, your mind will do what it can to make that true. You will shut down your brain's idea factory that could help you find a solution. Conversely, if you believe a solution is possible, your mind will help you find ways to make that true.

To turn negative thinking around, it's important to recognize when it occurs. Sometimes that critical voice in our heads is so prevalent that we take it to be the authority and forget to challenge it. If you find yourself having a negative thought, ask, "Is this true for me now?" Become your best friend and tell yourself only what you would say to your best friend.

According to Healthline.com (57), positive self-talk can:

- Increase vitality
- Give greater satisfaction with life
- Boost immune function
- Reduce pain
- Improve cardiovascular health
- Promote overall better physical well-being
- Lower the risk of death
- Reduce stress and distress

If you find that your thoughts are more shooting gallery than ticker-tape parade, following are a few ideas for changing that around.

Ways to Improve Mindset

Start a gratitude journal. Think of three to five things each day that you're grateful for. Write these down at the end of each day, making them your last thoughts as you drift off. Gratitude helps us re-experience something positive, doubling its impact. And training ourselves to acknowledge positive events rather than let them slip by unnoticed is great mindset training.

Connect with positive people. If you end up spending a lot of time with Negative Nancy, that's bound to affect you. If you need a reason to avoid negative people, remember that negative attitudes are contagious and that negative thoughts can impact your health and shorten your life. Choose to spend time with people who uplift you and support you, people who, after you've spent time with them, leave you with positive feelings and memories.

Find the humor in even bad situations. The Mayo Clinic reports that a good laugh has both short- and long-term benefits. (58) Short-term, it can stimulate your organs by enhancing your intake of oxygen. It stimulates your heart, lungs, and muscles, and increases the endorphins produced by your brain. It activates and relieves your stress response, decreasing your heart rate and blood pressure, and resulting in feelings of relaxation. Long-term, it can improve your immune system. Positive thoughts release neuropeptides that help fight stress and ward off illness. Laughter is also a pain reliever, and can enhance personal connections, increase feelings of happiness, and improve self-esteem.

Be positive about aging. Studies have shown that having a positive attitude about aging can prevent falls, ward off age-related illness and disease, and help us live longer.

Recall moments of triumph. Look back across your life and make a list. What challenges have you overcome? What have you done extremely well? What do you often receive compliments for? If learning to accept compliments is difficult, make it a practice to say, "Thank you" and internally, reaffirm, "This is true for me." Save any cards or notes or emails you receive from others that ring true to you and show you how awesome you really are. Review these if you begin to doubt yourself.

Affirmations

Optimists have a 19% lower mortality rate than pessimists, according to studies by the Mayo Clinic. (59) To turn your thinking more positive, spend time each day with positive affirmations. Choose those you can believe and that help you counter your most frequent negative self-talk. Write these yourself and recite them aloud. If that feels like too much work for now, try listening to one of the many positive affirmation videos on YouTube and putting those you like on Post-it notes throughout your home. Marcus Aurelius said, "When you arise in the morning, think of what a precious privilege it is to be alive—to breathe, to think, to enjoy, to love." Each day when you wake up, tell yourself it's going to be a wonderful day.

Your brain processes 60,000 thoughts per day. That's 35 to 42 thoughts per minute! How many of these are positive? If negative thinking is impacting you and you've been unable to turn it around, seek counseling. A mental health expert can help you address the "why" of your negative self-talk. This impacts everything, including your enjoyment of life, your health, and your longevity. Make it a priority.

Mindfulness

Mindfulness means noticing what's going on at any given moment without judgment. We may think we do this all the time, but much of our life is spent on autopilot. Mindfulness means being fully aware. What do you see, feel, hear? Mindfulness doesn't ask you to change your thinking or behavior in the moment, but simply to accept that this is how things are for you right now, without reacting. Being mindful allows you to see situations objectively and recognize that you have choices in how to respond. With mindfulness, you become an objective observer of your own life.

Reaction without mindfulness: "Brenda and Micah are so obnoxious. I can't stand being around them."

Reaction with mindfulness: "I'm noticing that I'm uncomfortable being around Brenda and Micah."

Become curious about a feeling. Don't judge, just notice. By not shutting down the feeling immediately, you can explore it.

"I think I'm envious. Do I wish my relationship were more like theirs?"

We miss so much of our own lives by not noticing the present moment. How often have you arrived somewhere and forgotten the journey? It's common for most of us to "tune out" our own lives and get wrapped in our thoughts of the future or the past, missing what's happening in the now. But the present moment *is* our life and we deserve to experience every moment of it.

What if you could view every event in your life as an objective observer, seeing it as an adventure leading to something new, rather than labeling the event as either good or bad? Zen Master Thich Nhat Hanh, known as the father of mindfulness, says, "The present moment is filled with joy and happiness. If you are attentive, you will see it."

At this very moment, I'm sitting in my bed with my laptop. A glass of Montepulciano d'Abruzzo is on my nightstand. My dog, Daisy, is curled up at the foot of my bed, her chest gently rising and falling. I can hear my son watching a video in the next room and traffic on the road a few blocks from my house. The soft light of my lamp spills across my comforter, fading into shadow at the other side of my bed. And I almost missed it.

Norman Lear titled his memoir *Even This I Get to Experience!* In it, he shares his lifelong practice of meeting each event in his life with a sense of wonder. When we slow down and focus on what's happening, we can appreciate the present moment and experience more joy and happiness in our lives—a goal worthy of a Goddess!

Ways to Increase Mindfulness

In the hurly-burly world of our lives, it can be difficult to remember to stop and take a breath. It may be helpful to begin at the start of your day. Take time each morning to have a few moments to yourself, to be thankful for a new day, and to be present. Avoid checking email, social media, or texts. Instead, give yourself your full attention. Check in with yourself. How are you feeling? What's on your mind?

When you eat breakfast or have coffee, do so mindfully, noticing tastes, temperatures, and textures. Take the time to chew each bite of food. Keep the cell phone off or away from the table.

Spend time in nature. Go for a walk around your neighborhood or visit a local park, trail, or greenspace. Observe the weather, the sights, the sounds, the smells.

Don't multitask. Multitasking has been found to be extremely inefficient. By dividing your attention, you're unable to give any moment, any task the attention it deserves. It may be hard to imagine getting into the Zen of dishwashing but let yourself experience it in a new way.

Be creative. If you have a creative hobby you enjoy, this provides a great opportunity to practice mindfulness. Experience the texture of the paint, clay, or cloth. See your hands moving over the items; notice how you create form from simple materials.

When you are more aware of each present moment, you will experience a richer, more fulfilling life.

Mindfulness through Meditation

There is no need for you to leave the house. Stay at your table and listen. Don't even listen, just wait. Don't even wait, be completely quiet and alone. The world will offer itself to you to be unmasked; it can't do otherwise; in raptures it will writhe before you. ~ Franz Kafka

A wonderful way to cultivate mindfulness is through meditation. Meditation is part of almost all forms of religion, and it's practiced by many atheists as well. Meditation is distinct from positive thinking. Positive thinking says, "This is great!" whereas meditation says, "This is." Meditation brings equanimity: mental calmness, composure, and evenness of temper, even in difficult situations. We could all use more of that, right?

A quote of unknown origin (often attributed to Mark Twain) goes, "In my life I have had many troubles, some of which actually happened." Worries, fears, and imagined catastrophes are simply the mind's way of protecting us from the worst possible outcomes. But living in fear diminishes us. Meditation helps us realize that we often mistake the stories we create for reality. This realization makes it possible to move toward greater sanity, well-being, and purpose.

Meditation isn't something you have to work to achieve; it's as close as your own breath. You simply follow your breath from the inhale through the exhale and repeat this process throughout the meditation session. Just a few breaths are all it takes to feel calmer. Even one minute a day (or several times a day) will reap many benefits.

When you meditate, you may be distracted by random thoughts. Some have equated trying to meditate to being crammed in a phone booth with a large crowd of people, all of whom are suffering from emotional disturbances. Here's the good news: Having distracting thoughts and noticing them *is* meditation! That's its entire purpose: to notice and release distracting thoughts. By noticing and releasing, you can clearly see that your thoughts are separate from you and that you control them versus them controlling you. That's worth the price of admission right there. You will soon see how often you're distracted by memories, thoughts, or fantasies about the past or future. Meditation isn't the cessation of thinking; it's training yourself to remember to come back to the present (the breath or some other focal point). Every part of this—the distraction, the noticing, the releasing—is meditation.

I credit Jeff Warren, a meditation teacher I discovered on the Calm app, for helping me demystify and simplify my meditation practice. I used to believe I couldn't meditate because I was unable to shut off what the Buddha calls the "monkey mind." I also used to be afraid that if I went "too deep" while meditating, I might not be able to come back. Now I know that these thoughts are incorrect and laughable, respectively. Meditation isn't about blanking out. It's about noticing thoughts without being controlled by them, just as if they were passing clouds. And as far as going too deep and not coming back, I doubt even transcendental meditators would be able to pull that off!

Like mindfulness, meditation is nonjudgmental awareness, and its purpose is both simple and profound. By realizing we're separate from our thoughts, we avoid knee-jerk reactions and can make better decisions, leading to a more peaceful life. Through meditation, we learn that we are not our monkey mind, but something far nobler, something Goddess-like.

The health benefits of meditation include reducing blood pressure, helping our bodies recover from cortisol spikes (caused by stress) improving our immune function response, slowing age-related brain atrophy, and lessening the symptoms of depression and anxiety. Meditation practice has been shown to reduce violent behavior in prisons, boost productivity in the workplace, and improve both the behavior and academic results of school children. Meditation can make permanent changes in our brains. Neuroscientists have found that meditation rewires the parts of the brain involved in self-awareness, compassion, and resiliency.

Meditation in Three Steps

If you want to distill mindfulness meditation to its purest form, it's this: sit, breathe, let go.

Step 1: Sit

Even among the simplest meditation steps (sit), there's flexibility. Although it's recommended to meditate sitting either in a chair or on a floor with a straight back, I often meditate in bed, either lying down or sitting up, resting against the headboard. Whatever position you choose, a straight spine can help you breathe more fully. And if you're worried you'll nod off, sitting will help you remain alert. You can close your eyes or allow your gaze to rest softly about three feet in front of you.

Step 2: Focus

Next, bring your full attention to your breath, following it with your mind as you inhale and exhale. Mentally travel with your breath, feeling the sensation as it enters and leaves your body. You may find it easier to quiet the mind to think "inhale" and "exhale" or "in" and "out" as you breathe. Others breathe in "peace" and breathe out "love." Breathe fully but naturally from the diaphragm or belly, not from the chest. Chest breathing is associated with rapid, stressful breathing. Diaphragm or belly breathing is deeper, more relaxing, and slower. A slow breath tells your nervous system that you are safe, allowing you to relax.

Step 3: Notice and Release

When thoughts intrude and you feel your mind wander away from your breathing, simply refocus without judgment. When you notice a thought, you may want to say in your mind "thinking" to acknowledge you've noticed the thought, but you're not giving it center stage in that moment. It doesn't matter how many times you have to redirect your focus during your meditation. In fact, the more practice you have redirecting your focus, the better you'll get at meditating. You simply can't get this wrong! Over time, you'll have fewer distractions, and yet you may find that on some days you experience more distracting thoughts than usual. This is natural and perfectly okay.

Arlene, an account executive at a public relations agency I once worked for, is the most serene person I've ever known. I never saw her ruffled, angry, or rushed, and she always wore a sunny smile. Just being in her presence was calming. In an agency meeting, with ideas and opinions flying back and forth, Arlene was mostly silent. When she did speak, it was always a thoughtful contribution that went directly to the heart of the matter and both synthesized and simplified the ideas of the others. Outside of work, Arlene taught yoga, which many consider an active form of meditation.

If you're finding it difficult to start a meditation practice, or you'd just like a nice getaway, consider signing up for a meditation retreat. Meditating with others is powerful and affirming and it will help you realize that the same struggles and doubts you have are shared by others. You'll also find compassion and support, and we could all use a little more of that in our lives, right? A spiritual mentor of mine who had been practicing meditation for more than 40 years and frequently led meditation groups always took at least one meditation retreat each year in which she was merely a participant. She found that it both renewed her and helped her in her daily practice.

Goddess Gift: Book Recommendations

Books on positive mindset:
- *The Power of Positive Thinking*, by Dr. Norman Vincent Peale
- *How to Stop Worrying and Start Living*, by Dale Carnegie
- *Success Through a Positive Mental Attitude* by Napoleon Hill and W. Clement Stone
- *The Power of Your Subconscious Mind* by Joseph Murphy
- *Excuses Begone!* by Dr. Wayne Dyer
- *Learned Optimism* by Martin E.P. Seligman
- *Even This I Get to Experience!* by Norman Lear

You can also find YouTube videos by searching "positive mindset"

Books on mindfulness and meditation:
- *Why Can't I Meditate?* by Nigel Wellings
- *Meditation for Your Life* by Robert Butera, Ph.D.
- *Meditation for Fidgety Skeptics* by Dan Harris
- *Success through Stillness* by Russell Simmons

Also search for YouTube videos on "meditation" and select the subject you'd like ("sleep," "positivity," etc.) and check out these apps: Calm, Headspace.

(57) Healthline. "Positive Self-Talk: Benefits and Techniques," October 17, 2018.
https://www.healthline.com/health/positive-self-talk.
(58) Mayo Clinic. "Stress Relief from Laughter? It's No Joke."
https://www.mayoclinic.org/healthy-lifestyle/stress-management/in-depth/stress-relief/art-20044456.
(59) Maruta, Toshihiko, Robert C. Colligan, Michael Malinchoc, and Kenneth P. Offord. "Optimists vs Pessimists: Survival Rate Among Medical Patients Over a 30-Year Period." Mayo
Clinic Proceedings 75, no. 2 (February 1, 2000): 140–43.
https://doi.org/10.4065/75.2.140.

CHAPTER NINE

THE GODDESS IN NATURE

COMING HOME

You didn't come into this world. You came out of it, like a wave from the ocean. You are not a stranger here. ~ Alan Watts

Before we started forming communities and building cities, we spent most of our evolutionary history in a close relationship with nature. Therefore, we have an innate love of natural settings and feel at peace there. When was the last time you spent quality time outdoors? If you have trouble remembering, you're not alone. The average American spends only 7% of their life outdoors. The average Brit fares only 0.5% better. Compare this to the average time spent in front of a screen (be it television, computer, or smart phone). For Americans, it's 35% of their day.

Spending more time in nature (and less time in front of a screen) can improve our overall well-being. According to ActiveHealth.sg, too much screen time can cause physical strain to our eyes and bodies, sleep deprivation, obesity, susceptibility to chronic health conditions, reduced brain power, lowered social skills, poor emotional judgment, and lowered self-esteem.

How much screen time is too much is a question with only subjective answers, but more time in nature is a prescription most of us would do well to fill. How much nature time is enough? Experts say that optimum physical and psychological benefits are realized when we spend at least 150 minutes per week outdoors, and this can be done all in one day or over several days.

Health Benefits of Nature

In a Pennsylvania hospital study, it was found that patients who underwent gallbladder surgery and had a view of nature in the hospital were shown to have less pain, fewer complications, and were able to be released sooner than those that faced buildings or walls. (60)

Harvard Health reports that patients who had spinal surgery and were exposed to natural light healed faster and reported less pain. (61)

A 2020 YouTube video by the University of Minnesota titled "Healing Power of Nature" notes that the therapeutic benefits associated with spending time in nature include reduced blood pressure, reduced heart rate, reduced muscle tension, and lowered production of stress hormones.

In a TEDx video, "Prescribing Nature for Health," pediatrician Nooshin Razani reports that when we spend time in nature, our breathing slows, our anxiety and depression are reduced, and our empathy rises. And after three days in nature, the pre-fontal cortex relaxes and resets, which helps us tap into our creative and productive brain power. Her clinic now prescribes nature outings as one of its therapies.

Walking is an excellent form of exercise. But while walks in both nature and urban life engage the mind, they do so in profoundly different ways. In a city, we must keep track of traffic, sounds, and signs. In nature, we don't have to analyze our environment in the same way. Instead, we can relax and simply bask in the beauty and peace around us. We can breathe fresh air. We can find our calm.

Nature Helps Our Brains

In a Finnish study, researchers found that merely sitting in nature made people feel psychologically restored, and when they walked in nature, that benefit was magnified. (62) The University of Michigan demonstrated that those who walked in nature scored 20% better on a memory test than those who walked in the city. (63) And in another study, researchers compared brain activity in participants who spent 90 minutes walking in a grassland area with oak trees and shrubs to those who'd walked along a traffic-heavy four-lane roadway. Those who'd had the nature walk had reduced activity in the area of the brain that's attributed to repetitive thought focused on negative emotions. (64)

Our levels of serotonin increase when we go outside. Serotonin helps with mood regulation and sleep. It reduces depression, regulates anxiety, heals wounds, maintains bone health, and helps control our bowel function. When our serotonin levels are normal, we feel happier, calmer, more focused, less anxious, and more emotionally stable.

Being in nature, or even viewing scenes of nature can reduce negative feelings, such as anger, fear, or stress, and replace them with pleasant feelings. Time in nature helps reduce anxiety and depression.

In one study in *Mind*, 95% of participants reported elevated moods after spending time outside, changing from depressed, stressed, and anxious to calm and balanced. (65) Other studies demonstrate that time in nature results in psychological well-being, meaningfulness, and vitality.

Spending time in nature also increases our ability to pay attention. Because we find nature interesting, we naturally focus on what we are experiencing. Like meditation, this focused attention refreshes our brain for new tasks. Children with ADHD show an improved attention span after spending time in nature. (66)

Natural Sounds

Even the sounds of nature, such as birds chirping, waves crashing, or a burbling stream can benefit our brain health. Studies have found that those who listened to nature sounds performed better on demanding cognitive tests than those who listened to urban sounds such as traffic and the noise of a busy coffee shop. (67)

Natural Light

Being outside in natural light can also reduce seasonal affective disorder (SAD), which afflicts some people during certain times of the year. And it can boost our exposure to the vitamin D in sunlight. The best times of day to get your dose of vitamin D without risking too much UVA exposure are two hours before noon and two hours after.

Natural Water

We are evolutionarily wired to find ease near water. Ancient civilizations often settled near water because there were fewer predators, increased visibility, and a more abundant food supply.

We also have an emotional connection to water. Think of how exhilarating it felt to run through a sprinkler as a child, or how it feels to dip our toes in the ocean, swim, stand under a waterfall, or even soak in a hot tub. Think of the emotional response we experience when we first spy a body of water, smell the air after a rain, or catch a whiff of the salty ocean air after a long time away. These feelings are separate from rational and cognitive responses. There's a visceral, emotional connection. In his book of the same name, marine biologist Wallace Nichols defines "blue mind" as "a meditative state characterized by calm, peacefulness, unity, and a sense of general happiness and satisfaction with life in the moment." (68)

Ways to Get More Nature

- Take a daily walk. This is good for your physical health as well as your emotional and mental health.
- Visit the beach or a body of water.
- Plan your vacations around natural surroundings.
- Go rock hunting.

- Go hiking or "forest bathing." Hug a tree. Get some exercise in nature.
- Go camping.
- Go sailing, boating, canoeing, kayaking, paddle boarding, surfing, or swimming.
- Go skiing or sledding.
- Join an outdoor group, such as the Explorer's Club, Sierra Club, or Mazamas.
- Join a forestry preservation society or adopt a local park.
- Attend outdoor concerts.
- Sunbathe.
- Take up gardening.
- Rent a lookout tower from the Forest Service. (This is how my parents spent their honeymoon.)
- Take up snorkeling or scuba diving.

Bring Nature Indoors

- Open your curtains and blinds. Open your windows and get fresh air for least 30 minutes each day.
- Add house plants to every room in your home.
- Add cut flowers to the rooms you spend the most time in.
- Start an indoor herb garden.
- Add an indoor fountain.
- Listen to soundscapes.
- Place plants or trees outdoors so you can see them from your windows.
- Install a bird feeder outdoors where you can see it.
- Choose nature scenes for artwork.
- Choose natural colors and textiles for décor.
- Find natural candles, wax melters, or diffusers, or make your own using essential oils such as pure orange or lavender.
- Collect rocks, seashells, beach glass, and pieces of driftwood and decorate your windowsills.
- When you meet a friend for coffee or a meal, walk there, and/or choose an outdoor table when weather permits.

Goddess Gifts: Plant Care and Easy-Care Plants

If, like me, you don't have a green thumb, here are some tips for plant care, and a list of some of the easiest plants to grow indoors. If you have pets or small children around, check for toxicity before purchase.

Indoor Plant Tips

- Most plants grow best in well-drained soil in an appropriately sized container.
- Most people overwater. Yellow leaves indicate overwatering. Don't water if the top half-inch to one inch of soil is moist. Drooping leaves likely mean underwatering.
- Brown tips on leaves may mean the humidity is too low or may be caused by salts in your tap water.
- You'll know it's time to repot your plant into a larger container if the roots are circling the inside of the container. The best time to repot is spring or summer. If you find that your plant has multiple stems, you can use this opportunity to divide the plant into multiple plants.
- Spring is also a good time to fertilize, but don't overdo it, or you'll burn the plant. Know the appropriate fertilizer for your plant. In general, flowering plants require a fertilizer with equal parts nitrogen, phosphorus, and potassium.
- Dust or spritz and wipe your plants regularly. Plants with hairy leaves (e.g., African violets) need dusting. Plants with smooth leaves can handle the water. Keeping the dust off helps the plant soak up more sunshine.
- Prune as needed in the fall.
- If plants attract pests, treat them appropriately, and if they contract a disease, remove and dispose of them to keep them from harming their green brothers and sisters.

Easy Indoor Plants

Aglaonemas: This is a lush plant that you'll often see in hallways or other out of the way places because it thrives in about every light condition except direct sun. Keep this one moist and water consistently.

Air plants: These flowering plants don't have roots, so they don't have to be potted in soil. They make great hanging plants because the air circulation helps them thrive.

Christmas cactus: My grandmother used to love to grow this plant. It produces pink or red flowers in early winter, hence the name. It prefers bright light, and pruning it after it blooms will help it stay bushy and full.

Dieffenbachia: The non-scientific name for this plant is "dumb cane," which is a terrible name for a beautiful plant. It prefers warmer temperatures, so avoid placing it near drafts or windows.

Dracaena Giganta: This is a bright, variegated plant that does best in low to medium light. Water only when the soil feels dry.

Hedgehog aloe: This plant should be placed in a sunny spot, and it can even be kept outside during the summer. It requires very little water. It's a kissing cousin to the aloe vera plant, which is also an excellent choice, with leaves that can be used for healing and skin moisturizing. Aloe vera also needs little water but prefers indirect sunlight and it can grow for years without the need to repot it.

Jade plant: This plant has thick, glossy leaves and can be seen growing to impressive proportions. It needs lots of sunlight. Allow the soil to completely dry out before watering, but water soon after.

Lucky bamboo: This plant can be grown in water, but once it has abundant roots, it should be planted in soil.

Monstera: Adaptable to most light conditions, moderately drought tolerant, low maintenance, and beautifully showy.

Philodendron heartleaf: This lovely plant thrives in indirect light and does not like bright sunlight. It does need consistent watering but is somewhat forgiving in this area.

Ponytail palm: It likes a sunny spot; even full sun is fine. Water occasionally.

Pothos (Epipremnum): If you're looking for a hardy trailing houseplant, look no further. This one is almost impossible to kill. Pruning it will keep it fuller, and the cutting can be placed in water to root, making this a plant that keeps on giving. These plants like to dry out between watering, but then want their water *now*. They are tolerant of all types of light conditions.

Sansevieria: These plants are often called "snake plants," and they don't need a lot of water, aren't sensitive to temperature changes, and don't require special care. They're also highly sought-after for their air-purifying properties.

Spider plant (Chlorophytum como sum): These plants produce babies, which hang off them, so you'll often see them grown in hanging baskets. Because their roots also grow abundantly, you may need to re pot every couple of years. When the babies send out roots, you can remove them from the mama plant and make more plants. These do best in bright, indirect sunlight but can tolerate low-light areas as well. Water the plant when the top two inches of soil are dry, and it will be a happy camper.

ZZ plant: This plant does best when it's almost completely ignored! It prefers to be kept fairly dry.

(60) "View Through a Window May Influence Recovery from Surgery." Text. The Center for Health Design, October 16, 2012. https://www.healthdesign.org/knowledge-repository/ view-through-window-may-influence-recovery-surgery.

(61) Harvard Health. "A Prescription for Better Health: Go Alfresco," October 12, 2010. https://www.health.harvard.edu/mind-and-mood/ a-prescription-for-better-health-go-alfresco.

(62) Tyrväinen, Liisa, Ann Ojala, Marjo Neuvonen, Katja Borodulin, and Timo Lanki. "[Health and well-being from forests - experience from Finnish research]." Sante Publique (Vandoeuvre-Les-Nancy, France) S1, no. HS (May 13, 2019): 249–56. https://doi.org/10.3917/spub.190.0249.

(63) Stenfors, Cecilia U. D., Stephen C. Van Hedger, Kathryn E. Schertz, Francisco A. C. Meyer, Karen E. L. Smith, Greg J. Norman, Stefan C. Bourrier, et al. "Positive Effects of Nature on Cognitive Performance Across Multiple Experiments: Test Order but Not Affect Modulates the Cognitive Effects." Frontiers in Psychology 10 (2019). https://www.frontiersin.org/article/10.3389/fpsyg.2019.01413.

(64) Bratman, Gregory N., J. Paul Hamilton, Kevin S. Hahn, Gretchen C. Daily, and James J. Gross. "Nature Experience Reduces

Rumination and Subgenual Prefrontal Cortex Activation." Proceedings of the National Academy of Sciences 112, no. 28 (July 14, 2015): 8567–72.
   https://doi.org/10.1073/pnas.1510459112.

(65) Mind Organization. (2007). Ecotherapy: The green agenda for mental health. UK: Mind Publications.

(66) Taylor, A., Kuo, F. (2008). Children with attention deficits concentrate better after walk in the park. Journal of Attention Disorders; 12 (5), 402-09.

(67) Luo, Jiutong, Minhong Wang, and Ling Chen. "The Effects of Using a Nature-Sound Mobile Application on Psychological Well-Being and Cognitive Performance Among University Students." Frontiers in Psychology 12 (2021).
   https://www.frontiersin.org/article/10.3389/fpsyg.2021.699908.

(68) Nichols, Wallace J, and C. Cousteau. Blue Mind: How Water Makes You Happier, More Connected and Better at What You Do, 2018.

CHAPTER TEN

GODDESSES CONNECT

MAKING FRIENDS FOR LIFE

You are a part of me I do not know yet. ~ Valarie Kaur

In *The Rabbit Effect*, (69) author Kelli Harding, MD, reports on a 1978 study of the relationship between high blood cholesterol and heart health using rabbits for test subjects. Scientists couldn't figure out why one group of rabbits fared so much better than others in the same study. After accounting for all other factors, they discovered that a particularly nurturing lab technician, who petted and stroked the rabbits as she fed them, made the difference between a healthy heart and a heart attack. Kindness and connection saved rabbit lives.

It turns out that this is not only true for rabbits. In fact, Ponce de Leon would have done better forming a few close friends instead of looking for the fountain youth because longevity experts now agree that the single biggest factor to living a long, healthy, and happy life is connectedness. It's more important than exercise, more important than not smoking, and more important than maintaining a healthy weight.

The "Roseto Effect" is named after a scientific study of the residents of Roseto, Italy, who had a 30-35% lower mortality rate than the residents in surrounding areas. After controlling for all other factors, researchers found that the outstanding sociality of the town was what led to the townspeople's significant lifespan. (70)

Living with someone—even a non-intimate roommate—can decrease mortality risk by 10-32%. Volunteerism decreases it by 22%. Combine a happy marriage with connected friendships and a feeling of belongingness, and the decrease in mortality risk climbs to 65%.

Today, however, loneliness is real. Losing friends to moves, divorce, death, and other life transitions occurs more frequently as we age. And it's getting worse. A study published by the *American Sociological Review* reported that the average American had three close friends in 1985, but by 2004, that number had shrunk to two, and over that same period, those reporting no close friends at all had jumped from 10% to 25%. (71) The damaging effects on our mental and physical health caused by loneliness led British Prime Minister Theresa May to appoint a Minister of Loneliness. Manitoba also has a minister responsible for helping seniors stay socially engaged.

As we all know from the recent pandemic, social isolation is sometimes mandated for health reasons. On top of this, race wars and political divisions are causing family rifts and distrust of our neighbors. But even if all of that weren't going on, connections tend to decrease as we age. During our teen years, one-third of our time is spent with friends. For the rest of our lives, it's less than 10%. In *Love Your Age*, author Barbara Hannah Grufferman cites the following contributing factors to fewer meaningful connections. (72)

- Decreasing engagement (lower religious participation, fewer connections in the workplace, a reduction in civic participation)
- Busyness and time pressure (Time with our friends is often the first thing we cross off our schedules.)
- Economic hard times
- Residential mobility
- Television and gadgetry
- Disruption of marriage and family ties
- Growth of the welfare state
- Cultural revolt against authority

While it may take effort on our part to establish connections as we age, given the huge rewards, it's worth the effort. In her 2019 book, *The*

Positive Shift: Mastering Mindset to Improve Happiness, Health, and Longevity, author Catherine A. Sanderson writes, "The single biggest predictor of our happiness is the quality of our relationships." (73) She stresses having meaningful conversations, not merely chit chat, and says that even a brief meaningful conversation, such as a moment of human connection in an exchange with a store clerk, increases our feelings of belongingness and happiness.

Kenzoku and Ubuntu

Tom Roth, a Gallup researcher, studied the homeless to find out why they were living on the streets. One commonality? A lack of healthy friendships. He asked this question as a determining factor: "Who expects you to be somebody?" For many of the homeless, the answer was "No one." (74)

There are two words to keep in mind when seeking to increase connectedness: *kenzoku* and *ubuntu. Kenzoku* is the Japanese term for people in our lives who are committed to our happiness and wellbeing. It means family, but not necessarily those who are blood related. In Richard Bach's book, *Illusions: The Adventures of a Reluctant Messiah*, he writes "The bond that links your true family is not one of blood, but of respect and joy in each other's life. Rarely do members of one family grow up under the same roof." (75) Fred Rogers, of Mr. Rogers fame, loved the South African word *ubuntu*, which means "I am because you are. My identity is such that it includes you. I would be a very different person without you."

Who expects you to be somebody? How many connections do you feel *kenzoku* or *ubuntu* with? And what is the optimum number? Believe it or not, there is one: four. In a 2001 Duke University study (cited in *The Positive Shift*) analyzing 400 patients, researchers found that those who had at least four close friends lived significantly longer than others, even when controlling for all other variables. Four was the magic number—more didn't increase longevity benefits. However, the quality of our friendships matters even more than the quantity. It's better to have two close friends than 100 acquaintances.

Friends play many roles in our lives, and usually, one person—even a partner or spouse you consider your soulmate—can't fulfill all these roles. In *Vital Friends,* Roth listed eight essential roles:

- **Builder:** Someone who motivates you to succeed and is a catalyst for your personal and professional growth
- **Champion:** A person who sings your praises to others and stands up for you even when you're not around
- **Collaborator:** Someone with interests and passions like your own
- **Companion:** Someone who is always there for you and thinks nothing of sacrificing for your benefit, a lifetime friendship
- **Connector:** A bridge builder who introduces you to others and furthers your course; a person who seems to know everyone
- **Energizer:** A fun friend who gives you a boost and makes you laugh
- **Mind Opener:** Someone who encourages you to think in innovative ways and broadens your perspective on life
- **Navigator:** This person provides guidance, helps you with decision making, and helps you find clarity

There will be some crossover, and as the Duke University study suggests, there's no reason to strive for eight close friends when four will do; some people will serve more than one role. And you may find that someone who is not actually a friend is serving one of the roles. For instance, a therapist may fill the Navigator role. The purpose of identifying the primary roles your friends play is that it gives you a focus area for deepening your connection. Sharpen this area. Focus on what's already working well.

Deepening Existing Friendships

Emerson said, "The only way to have a friend is to be one." If you would like to have more meaningful connection in your life, what efforts are you making? For women, gender is on our side. Women are biologically adapted to help each other through challenging times. When a woman is stressed, estrogen helps her body release oxytocin, which stops the fight or flight stress reaction and causes her to seek nurturing contact.

During this contact, the body releases even more oxytocin, which increases the calming effect. Men, on the other hand, have higher levels of testosterone, especially when under stress, and testosterone reduces the effects of oxytocin.

To create closeness in a friendship requires only two steps: increase your understanding of one another (knowingness) and increase your investment in each other's well-being (caring). In *Stop Being Lonely*, author Kira Asatryan writes, "A long-term relationship requires regular participation in the act of knowing and caring." (76) To get to **know** someone better, she advises:

- Have deeper conversations
- Find unifying commonalities while accepting your differences
- Talk productively about the past and the future (whining is an energy drain)
- Comfortably disclose your inner world
- Meet in person
- Ask deeper questions (For instance, if a friend says she likes a particular author's books, ask her what she likes about them.)

To deepen the **caring** aspect of your friendship (or check to see whether your friendships are deeply connected), Asatryan advises that you:

- Feel and identify emotions
- Be empathetic
- Bond without losing your identity
- Show someone explicitly that you care (as an example, I've recently begun to tell people for whom this is true, 'You can call me any time, day or night, for any reason.')
- Handle disagreements while still communicating in a caring way
- Maintain the bond of caring over time
- Respond appropriately (hold a hand when expressing concern)
- Take responsibility as appropriate (apologize sincerely)
- Be able to accept caring

Forming New Friendships

Okinawans have one of the world's largest percentages of centenarians. Okinawans live by the motto *ichariba choade*, which means "Treat everyone like a brother, even if you've never met."

In one of my favorite movies, *American Dreamer*, starring JoBeth Williams and Tom Conti, the lead character, Kathy, a stay-at-home mom with a less-than-supportive husband, enters a writing contest to win a trip to Paris. When she returns home after running errands, carrying groceries and dry cleaning, she trips and falls inside the front door where she spies a telegram that had been slipped through her mail slot. Still on the floor, she closes her eyes, crosses her fingers, opens the envelope, and extracts the telegram, then opens her eyes to finally read that she has won the contest. This is a pivotal moment in her dreary life. Beside herself with joy, she looks around for someone to tell. But there is no one. "I won!" she mouths, wordlessly. "I won!"

Sharing life's wins is just as important as sharing its sorrows. When something pivotal happens in our lives, it's only natural to reach out to a friend to share it with. Joys are doubled; burdens are halved when shared. But what if, like Kathy, no one springs to mind? It's time to form new friendships. One or two new close friends is a great starting goal.

The Stigma of Loneliness

There is no shame in loneliness—but there is great sadness in failing to do something about it. The need for friends has somehow become stigmatized. In *The Friendship Crisis,* author Marla Paul writes that somehow "It's perfectly acceptable to be on the prowl for a man or a partner, but don't go announcing to the world that you're looking for a friend. Women fear we have some glaring personal flaw if we're not flanked by companions." (77)

One reason it's often hard to find new companions is that no one realizes that other people are looking, too! Loneliness is universal, but it's not incurable. I used to dread parties where I knew few, if any, people. But now, if I find myself in a roomful of strangers, I look for the person standing alone. I approach this person and introduce myself. They're usually so relieved that someone is talking to them that it's a successful encounter. We start with small talk, and the conversation deepens over time. Then, when someone approaches or passes nearby, looking lost, I introduce both of us to the newcomer. This is a formula that always works. By helping others with their loneliness, suddenly you're surrounded by a crowd.

But ... What If I'm Shy?

The first step in overcoming shyness is liking yourself. If people sense you're uncomfortable it can be off-putting. So, like yourself and learn to be comfortable with your shyness. Most people appreciate a shy person; their reserve is a refreshing alternative to those who monopolize conversations, bulldoze everyone in their path, and seem to shout "Me, me, me!" with every word.

Another tip is to be genuinely interested in others. The people we like best are the ones who are interested in us. Consider yourself a reporter whose job it is to get the story. Everyone has one. Focusing on the stories of others and demonstrating genuine interest in them will help you recognize commonalities, and you'll find yourself naturally more at ease in sharing your own story.

Too Busy for Friends?

As Paul writes in *The Friendship Crisis*, what separates busy women who have time for friends from those who don't is attitude. They make time for their friends. They "spackle them into the cracks in their lives." In other words, women who form, deepen, and preserve their shifting friendships work at it.

As we've already discussed, multitasking is overrated, but it can be a beneficial way to stay in touch with friends when time is short. Here are some options:
- Work out together, either at the gym on by going for a walk
- Meet for coffee or breakfast early before work
- Meet for lunch

- Take a class together
- Invite a friend for dinner
- Use a headset on your phone while chatting with your friend and doing household chores
- Run errands together
- Schedule spa days or beauty treatments together

Make sure to schedule your next get-together before you part. Standing appointments with friends are also great ways to stay in touch. I have four groups of friends I have standing meetings with. These may give you ideas for forming your own regular connections:

- A Mastermind group: We meet weekly on Thursdays at 6 a.m.
- A writing partner: We meet Saturdays at a coffee shop and write in tandem for two hours.
- Work colleagues, a group called The Resigning Women. In addition to participating in a private Facebook group, we meet monthly for a virtual happy hour.
- Women and Wine: This formed out of a Meetup group, and it's a new group for me, but I'm enjoying the interaction. We meet monthly for wine and conversation, sometimes virtually, sometimes in person.

All these connections are a huge part of the satisfaction and happiness I feel in my life. When I think of my life's blessings, warm connections are right at the top!

Organizations That May Help

A great way to meet new friends is to participate in Meetups and volunteer activities that interest you. When I lived on Maui for two years, I formed a beach clean-up Meetup group and made several friends that way. One couple I met through that Meetup group invited my son and me for dinner at their Maui condominium, and because they lived permanently in Oregon (my home state), when my son and I moved back, we've been able to stay in touch.

Besides Meetup, here are a few organizations that may help you form new friendships: widownet.org, griefnet.org, parentswithoutpartners.

org, divorcecare.org, home-based working moms (mbwm.com), work at home moms (wahm.com), and mothersandmore.org.

As I learned when I moved to Maui in 2015, breaking into a new community is often agonizingly slow. To ease the transition, seek out other newcomers and join women's groups and clubs within the groups. When someone says, "Let's get together and do X sometime," pin them down. If they're unwilling to commit, it may not be worth pursuing. Knock on a neighbor's door and introduce yourself. Check your church, synagogue, or community center for a friendship or discussion group. Inquire about book clubs at your local library or bookstore or start one. A book club I began nearly 20 years ago is still going strong.

Consider these other ideas for places to meet new friends:

- A memoir writing class
- Newcomersclub.org
- American Association for University Women (aauw.org)
- Boot camps and other exercise classes
- Walking your dog or volunteering to walk your neighbor's dog.

Before spending money on a membership fee, see if you can participate in an activity or two. Give it two or three chances before giving up. And be sure they hold activities! For instance, I joined a national society, and after paying my membership fee, I found out that my local chapter hadn't held an event in ages.

Want to track down old friends? One useful source is classmates.com.

Recognizing a Friend

Not everyone you meet will become your friend, and there will be times when someone wants to be your friend, but you don't want to be theirs. Let them know sooner than later. I once met a woman who desperately wanted to be my friend. She was aggressive in her friendship advances, making plans for us without asking me and not wanting to take no for an answer. That was bad enough, but she also swore incessantly, was incredibly angry, and played the victim about every relationship, job, or friendship she'd ever had. On top of all of that, she had an annoying habit of sitting too close and poking me with her finger whenever she wanted to emphasize a point. After making excuses a few times about why I couldn't get together with her, I finally had to be direct. "I'm sorry, we are in two different places in our lives, and I don't think this friendship is going to work out. But I wish you every happiness." She took it better than I expected, not that she had much choice—I was firm. This lifted a huge weight off my shoulders! If you find yourself dreading the time you spend with someone (or feeling like you need a salt scrub, smudging, or exorcism after you do), it's time for some tough love and the firm closing of a door. This will make room for the friends you do want in your life.

On the other hand, a potential friend may not look like you expect. For instance, he or she may be much older or much younger than you. That's a wonderful thing! Think how much you can learn from one another. I have friends who are 20 years younger than me, and I've had friends who've been 30 years older than me. A friend may also be from a different culture, race, or economic class. If the elements of true friendship are there, this shouldn't matter. To recognize a potential friend, ask yourself:

Do you feel like she's really listening to you, or does she just want to talk about herself?

I nearly gave up a friend because she was constantly talking about herself. I found that if I made sure she knew she was heard, I could add relevant commentary, and she was genuinely interested in hearing my stories, too. I think she had felt responsible for keeping both ends of the conversation going. When I finally chimed in with my "two cents," she seemed surprised and relieved that I had something to say! Our conversations are never going to be 50/50, but I think we're both more comfortable now that we're at least 70/30.

Can she accept your thoughts and feelings without judging or criticizing you?

I've been fortunate—or simply proactive—in avoiding people like this. A friend who criticizes and judges is no friend at all.

Does she share information about herself or is it one-sided?

I've had friends who were very willing to listen to everything I had to say but shared little of themselves. I would find out later that something monumental had occurred in their life, and it hadn't been shared with me. That's hurtful. When this occurs, ask yourself, "Am I showing this person that I'm truly interested in her life?" If you are, and that person is still not sharing, it's possible that person will never be a close friend. True friendship is reciprocal.

Does she gossip or spill others' confidences or criticize them behind their backs?

Chances are she'll do the same to you.

How to Be a Friend

Friendship requires effort and it requires time. If you have a spouse or partner who's uncomfortable with the idea of you spending time with your friends, explain why your friendship time is important to you, and that your partner will benefit because it will make you a happier person. If that fails, ask why it's an issue. Offer to alternate weekly guys' nights for a gals' night out. Don't ask for permission; announce your intentions. This is for your health, your happiness, and your longevity. And all of that can aid your relationship with your partner.

Friends make time for one another. To be a friend, schedule time together. Also:

- Pay attention/listen with both ears (Don't be thinking about what you want to say and don't interrupt.)
- Be kind—to me, this is the minimum requirement in any friendship.
- Stay in touch and don't worry about whose turn it is!
- Celebrate successes—yes, even if you're envious or jealous!
- Rain compliments—we all like to receive genuine compliments.
- Show up for happy and sad events—weddings, birthdays, recitals, funerals.
- Remember birthdays and anniversaries.
- If something is important to you, say so. Don't make your friend guess, then act hurt because she forgot.
- Give a gift for no special reason. Around the holidays a few years ago, two friends from two areas of my life sent me photos of gifts I'd given them more than 20 years earlier. They'd saved the gifts all that time and were somehow both prompted to let me know how much the items had meant to them. For reference, these were handmade

gifts that cost me very little but my time and creativity, and they included photos of the two of us spending time together as friends.
- Return calls and emails promptly—and take those calls even if you have to say, "Is it important? If not, can I call you back in a half-hour?" And then follow through.
- Accept their imperfections (frequently late, etc.).
- Accept their apologies. I once lost a dear friend of many years who was upset about my take on a situation. It was just a miscommunication, but I had inadvertently offended her, and no amount of my apologizing made any difference! I tried phone calls, letters, and texts and finally gave up. Sometimes friendship runs its course, and we must accept it. (But darn, it hurts!)
- Pitch in when help is needed. Don't wait to ask, "What can I do?" Just do it.

For Further Reading

Improving our connections is vital. I hope this chapter has inspired you to deepen existing friendships and form new ones. If you'd like to do further reading on this subject, I've mentioned several books already that are good starting points. I'll list them again here, plus a few others I found helpful as I was researching this important topic.

50 is the New Fifty: Ten Life Lessons for Women in Second Adulthood by Suzanne Braun Levine

Frientimacy: How to Deepen Friendships for Lifelong Health and Happiness by Shasta Nelson

Growing Young: How Friendship, Optimism, and Kindness Can Help You Live to 100 by Marta Zaraska

How to Create a Mastermind Group: The Power Hour Ticket to Everything You've Ever Wanted by Cicely Maxwell

How to Make Friends as an Adult: Advice to Help You Expand Your Social Circle, Nurture Meaningful Relationships, and Build a Healthier, Happier Social Life by Hope Kelaher

How to Start a Conversation and Make Friends by Don Gabor

Love Your Age: The Small-Step Solution to a Better, Longer, Happier Life by Barbara Hannah Grufferman

Madly in Love with Me: The Daring Adventure of Becoming Your Own Best Friend by Christine Arylo

Stop Being Lonely: Three Simple Steps to Developing Close Friendships and Deep Relationships by Kira Asatryan

The Friendship Crisis: Finding, Making, and Keeping Friends When You're not a Kid Anymore by Marla Paul

The Positive Shift: Mastering Mindset to Improve Happiness, Health, and Longevity by Catherine A. Sanderson

The Rabbit Effect: Live Longer, Happier, and Healthier with the Groundbreaking Science of Kindness by Kelli Harding, MD

The Relationship Cure: 5 Step Guide to Strengthening Your Marriage, Family, and Friendships by John M. Gottman, PhD and Joan DeClaire

Vital Friends: The People You Can't Afford to Live Without by Tom Rath

Goddess Gift: Friendship Quotes

Following are a few quotes on friendship that you may want to add to a note or gift to a friend, or just to inspire you.

"I would rather walk with a friend in the dark, than alone in the light." ~ Helen Keller

"A good friend knows all your stories. A best friend helped you create them." ~ Unknown

"A friend is someone who makes it easy to believe in yourself."~ Heidi Wills

"Rare as is true love, true friendship is rarer." ~ Jean de La Fontaine

"Some people arrive and make such a beautiful impact on your life, you can barely remember what life was like without them." ~ Anna Taylor

"Many people will walk in and out of your life, but only true friends will leave footprints in your heart." ~ Eleanor Roosevelt

"I knew when I met you an adventure was going to happen." ~ Winnie The Pooh

"Friendship is born at that moment when one person says to another: 'What! You too? I thought I was the only one.'" ~ C.S. Lewis

"Friendship is always a sweet responsibility, never an opportunity." ~ Khalil Gibran

"It's the friends you can call up at 4 a.m. that matter." ~ Marlene Dietrich

"The great thing about new friends is that they bring new energy to your soul." ~ Shanna Rodriguez

"Close friends are truly life's treasures. Sometimes they know us better than we know ourselves. With gentle honesty, they are there to guide and support us, to share our laughter and our tears. Their presence reminds us that we are never really alone." ~ Vincent Van Gogh

"You can always tell when two people are best friends because they're always having way more fun than it makes sense for them to be having." ~ Unknown

"Anything is possible when you have the right people there to support you." ~ Misty Copeland

"There is nothing I would not do for those who are really my friends." ~ Jane Austen

"Surround yourself with only people who are going to lift you higher." ~ Oprah Winfrey

(69) Harding, Kelli. The Rabbit Effect: Live Longer, Happier, and Healthier with the Groundbreaking Science of Kindness. New York: Atria Books, 2019.

(70) Egolf, B, J Lasker, S Wolf, and L Potvin. "The Roseto Effect: A 50-Year Comparison of Mortality Rates." American Journal of Public Health 82, no. 8 (August 1992): 1089–92.

https://www.ncbi.nlm.nih.gov/pmc/articles/PMC1695733/.

(71) "Americans Have Fewer Friends Outside the Family, Duke Study Shows."

https://today.duke.edu/2006/06/socialisolation.html.

(72) Grufferman, Barbara Hannah. Love Your Age: The Small-Step Solution to a Better, Longer, Happier Life. Washington, D.C: National Geographic, 2018.

(73) Sanderson, Catherine Ashley. The Positive Shift: Mastering Mindset to Improve Happiness, Health, and Longevity. Dallas, TX: BenBella Books, 2019.

(74) Rath, Tom. Vital Friends: The People You Can't Afford to Live Without. New York, NY: Gallup Press, 2006.

(75) Bach, Richard. Illusions: The Adventures of a Reluctant Messiah. New York: Bantam, 1989.

(76) Asatryan, Kira. Stop Being Lonely: Three Simple Steps to Developing Close Friendships and Deep Relationships. Novato, California: New World Library, 2016.

(77) Paul, Marla. The Friendship Crisis: Finding, Making, and Keeping Friends When You're Not a Kid Anymore. Pennsylvania: Rodale, 2006.

CHAPTER ELEVEN

GODDESS DREAMS AND GOALS

GIVING WINGS TO YOUR DREAMS

Do not fear to be your true self. Everything you want, wants you.
~ Genevieve Behrend

Growth, another word for personal development, is the Goddess way. It's foundational for a life well lived. Personal development fosters better relationships, reduces stress, benefits our health, increases productivity, helps us self-regulate, breeds success, makes us more resilient, and increases feelings of contentment and happiness. Yet Americans spend far more on the beauty treatments and products than they do on self-improvement. Blame it on the Kardashians.

Growth can feel scary at times. When we attempt something new, we have to forge a new trail to get there. Every step is new, so time appears to stretch out. It's taking forever. The pull to give up is real. This is natural, and we must overcome it to achieve anything new. Many years ago, I read *The Artist's Way* by Julia Cameron. (78) The book was a phenomenon at the time of its publication, and I still highly recommend it. As much as I loathe in-book exercises, those in *The Artist's Way* challenge you and help you unleash your creativity, not in a *let's-all-make-macrame-plant-hangers* way, but in expanding your life in new, exciting ways.

One exercise designed to uncover submerged dreams and goals follows. If you're up for it, quickly, without censoring yourself, write down five answers to each of the following:

1. Hobbies that sound like fun
2. Classes that sound like fun
3. Activities you personally would never do that sound like fun
4. Skills that would be fun to have
5. Activities you used to enjoy doing
6. Silly things you would like to try once

While five may seem like a lot, it requires you to dig deeper, which is often where the goals and desires live that excite you the most.

Here's an exercise that I developed as an alternative.

Imagine you're interviewing for a position with your eight-year-old self. She wants to see how her life would turn out if she employed you to be her older self. Would she approve of where you are now? Of the career path you've chosen? The adventures you've had? Your relationships? Your health? Remember, she's rooting for you to get the job! What changes would you need to make to ensure your eight-year-old self would be excited to be you when she grows up?

You deserve to make both your eight-year-old self and your current self happy and proud. You are a Goddess, and like most Goddesses, you've probably been taking care of responsibilities and people—family, friends, and lovers—while ignoring your own dreams and interests. When might be a good time for you to change that?

Living the Dream

What postponed dream can you make true for yourself today? This week? This year? Pick at least one dream that really excites you.

If your thoughts automatically go to excuses for why you can't, here are a few Goddess cures from the experts.

Excuse: I'm too old.

Cure: No, you're not. Let Dear Abby tell you why in an oft-requested column.

DEAR ABBY: I am a 36-year-old college dropout whose lifelong ambition was to be a physician. I have a very good job selling pharmaceutical supplies, but my heart is still in the practice of medicine. I do volunteer work at the local hospital on my time off, and people tell me I would have made a wonderful doctor.

If I go back to college and get my degree, then go to medical school, do my internship, and finally get into the actual practice of medicine, it will take me seven years! But, Abby, in seven years I will be 43 years old. What do you think? — UNFULFILLED IN PHILLY

DEAR UNFULFILLED: And how old will you be in seven years if you don't go to medical school? (79)

We get this one precious life, and it can be, as Hellen Keller said, either a daring adventure or nothing at all. What adventure will you dare to take?

Excuse: It costs too much.

Goddess Cure: Too much for what?

The value of something is what it's worth to you. If your dream is important to your self-worth or your satisfaction in life, how much is too much? Try brainstorming ways to raise the funds. What can you let go of to cover the costs? Can you get a scholarship for it, or is there another way to obtain it at a reduced or free cost? Let's say you wanted to spend a year abroad. Can you rent out your house to cover most of your expenses? Can you hire yourself out as a traveling companion?

This dream you want is an investment in you. What cost is too dear?

Excuse: I'm too busy.

Goddess Cure: Affirm: There is always enough time to do what's meant for me.

Annie Dillard wrote, "How we spend our days is how we spend our lives." (80) Is your time being spent to bring you the life you want to live? If not, look for a way to free up your schedule to make room for your dreams. Try eliminating, delegating, or hiring out a low-value task for your higher value goal or dream.

Excuse: It's impossible.

Goddess Cure: Have others done it? Then why not you?

Napoleon Hill, author of the 1937 book *Think and Grow Rich*, wrote "Whatever your mind can conceive and believe, it can achieve." (81) Look at that word: "impossible." Notice how it parses out to:

I

M

Possible

Excuse: It's never been done before.

Goddess Cure: Someone has to be the first. Why not you?

In 1954, Roger Bannister broke the four-minute barrier for running a mile. Prior to 1954, all the experts said that it could not be done because the human body was not capable of running that fast. Others tried and failed. Bannister, too, had trained relentlessly and failed. But once he broke that barrier, running the mile in 3:59.4, less than a year later, another runner also ran the mile in under four minutes. And after that, the record was beaten 18 times more. The current record, set by Hicham El Guerrouj of Morocco in 1999, is 3:43.13, a full 15 seconds faster than Sir Roger. How long will it stand?

Excuse: I'm not prepared (Or: I don't know enough about it).

Goddess Cure: You don't have to see the whole highway. You just have to see far enough to take the next step.

You can prepare by researching and asking people who've been successful at it for their advice on how to get started. They're usually more than happy to mentor you.

And sometimes, luck favors the unprepared.

In 1983, a 61-year-old Australian sheep herder named Cliff Young entered one of the toughest ultra-marathons in the world. The event was a 543.7-mile (875-kilometer) endurance course from Sydney to Melbourne. To complete the run, participants needed to be able to run 18 hours every day, which left time for only six hours of sleep each night.

Elite athletes from all over the world entered. Cliff showed up at the starting line in his overalls and work boots. Everyone laughed. Cliff told anyone who asked why he had entered that he believed he had a fair chance, given that he grew up on a farm where he often had to round up the sheep without the help of a horse or tractor.

The race began, and Cliff ran in a slow, plodding shuffle. After the first few miles, he trailed badly at the back of the pack. By the second day, he was faring a bit better, and he continued to gain in position as the race progressed. By the last night, no one was laughing. Cliff had crossed the finish line first, setting a new world record. No one had told Cliff to sleep, so, he didn't.

He also didn't know there was a $10,000 award for the winner, and he refused it, instead having it split among his fellow runners. Elite athletes now train not to sleep on this run, and the "Young Shuffle" is a recognized gait used by runners to conserve energy in long-distance races.

Excuse: I don't know where to start.

Goddess Cure: Take the tiniest step and momentum will build. Action is on your side because it creates momentum.

"Until one is committed there is hesitancy, the chance to draw back, always ineffectiveness. Concerning all acts of initiative (and creation), there is one elementary truth, the ignorance of which kills countless ideas and splendid plans: that the moment one definitely commits oneself, then Providence moves too. All sorts of things occur to help one that would never otherwise have occurred. A whole stream of events issues from the decision, raising in one's favor all manner of unforeseen incidents and meetings and material assistance, which no man [or Goddess!] could have dreamed would have come [her] way." ~William Hutchinson Murray (1913-1996), The Scottish Himalayan Expedition

To begin, begin. As Johann Wolfgang von Goethe wrote, "Boldness has genius, power and magic in it."

Excuse: I'm afraid.

Goddess Cure: Fear is frozen fun.

It's okay to be afraid; in fact, it's almost a requirement for growth. As Jack Canfield said, "Everything you want is on the other side of fear." Try this: When you're inspired to do X, count down backward from five: *five, four, three, two, one*, and at "one" just do it. Or follow Eleanor Roosevelt's advice: "Do one thing every day that scares you." By taking risks and not having a piano fall on your head, you'll learn to take more risks. You'll become more comfortable with discomfort. And here's advice from Rosa Parks, *"I have learned over the years that when one's mind is made up, this diminishes fear; knowing what must be done does away with fear."* Visualize success on the other side of fear, know your plan, and execute it. Remember that our thoughts often go to the worst possible outcome to try to protect us from catastrophe, but there are no tigers chasing you. Nick Vujicic, author of *Life Without Limits*, recommends that we think of fear as an acronym: False Evidence Appearing Real. (82) Vujicic was born without arms or legs and is now an internationally renowned motivational speaker on finding life's purpose.

Excuse: I'll fail.

Goddess Cure: Maybe. At first. And that's great! Reach for the moon. As Norman Vincent Peale said, "Reach for the moon. Even if you fail, you'll land amongst the stars." The first step toward being good at anything is totally sucking at it. If baby birds gave up after their first attempts at flight, we'd have a lot of tiny penguins. Perseverance trumps early failure every time.

Excuse: They'll say no.

Goddess Cure: What will they say if you don't ask?

The answer to the unasked question is always no. But suppose you do get a "no" from whoever "they" are? It happens. People are resistant to change, and "no" can stop most people in their tracks. But that shouldn't stop you. Let them know you're serious. Ask again in another way, and another. If you continue to get a "no," there are always ways to get around, under, over, or through that no. Take that "no" as a chance to be creative. There may be another approach that will get you what you're after that you hadn't thought of.

Once, after being shown by my employer that I was three times as productive as my peers, I lobbied for a raise. I was told no. I reminded my employer of my stats. Again, I was told no. I then connected with a well-known thought leader in the same industry as my company, explaining my dilemma. She shared a story with me. "Several times I asked for a raise from my employer, to no avail. I finally had to leave the company to be paid what I was worth. Every single person they tried to hire to fill my vacancy wanted more money than I'd been asking for." I included that quote, attributed to her, on the last page of a PowerPoint presentation I prepared. And I got my raise.

A Message of Love

My friend, Sarah Love, is owner of I Stand for Love (istandforlove.com), an uplifting, love-based, indescribably yummy company that has been publishing an I Stand for Love calendar for nearly 20 years. You can sign up for daily love bombs in your email (a great way to start your day) and she will never spam you. As I was writing this book, one of her daily messages came and I knew it was a perfect inclusion for this chapter.

> Numbers don't even exist that come close to what your life is worth. You are irreplaceable. Beyond precious and unique. Not only are you worthy of Love and health and joy, your worth is off the charts. Take some time today to think about that. Feel it in your cells. There is only one you in the entire Universe. How rare and special you are!

How to Get Started

Your dreams matter and you deserve to have them come true. Arthur Ashe said, "Start where you are. Use what you have. Do what you can." Take the first step. If you need some encouragement, check out the quotes in your Goddess Gift for this chapter.

Rock on, Goddess! Lift your voice. The choir needs you.

Goddess Gift: Empowering Quotes

"We should all start to live before we get too old. Fear is stupid. So are regrets." ~ Marilyn Monroe

"None of us are getting out of here alive, so please stop treating yourself like an afterthought. Eat the delicious food. Walk in the sunshine. Jump in the ocean." ~ Richard Gere

"A year from now you may wish you had the momentum of starting today." ~ Karen Lamb

"Success requires first expending 10 units of effort to produce one unit of results. Your momentum will then produce 10 units of results with each unit of effort." ~ Charles J. Givens

"It's never too late to be who you might have been." ~ George Eliot

"A ship is safest when it is in port, but that's not what ships were built for." ~ Paulo Coelho

"Be patient with yourself. Self-growth is tender; it's holy ground. There's no greater investment." ~ Stephen Covey

"When a woman rises up in glory, her energy is magnetic and her sense of possibility contagious." ~ Marianne Williamson

Bonus: Goddess Adventure Options

Travel

- Travel and learn or travel and volunteer through one of these organizations:
- RoadScholar.org (educational trips for ages 50+)
- GlobalVolunteers.org (one- to three-week opportunities)
- GlobeAware.org (volunteer vacations)

Lifelong Learning

Self-paced online learning is known as eLearning. The global eLearning market is predicted to reach $325 billion by 2025, tripling its 2015 levels. Search online for courses of your interest, starting here.

- Seniorplanet.org has virtual classes for ages 60+
- Colleges throughout the U.S. have audit-only or credit options for some courses for a reduced or fee or free fee for seniors of varying ages.

E-books are available at your local library (as well as the paperback and hardback kind!)

- Language classes are available through Pimsleur, Babbel, Mondly, Rocket Languages, Rosetta Stone, Lingopie, and others

(78) Cameron, Julia. The Artist's Way: A Spiritual Path to Higher Creativity. 25th anniversary edition. New York, New York: TarcherPeregree, 2016.

(79) Chicago Tribune. "YOU'RE NEVER TOO OLD TO DO WHAT YOU LOVE."

https://www.chicagotribune.com/news/ ct-xpm-1994-12-27-9412270200-story.html.

(80) Dillard, Annie. The Writing Life. 1. ed., 11. print. New York, NY: HarperPerennial, 1995.

(81) Hill, Napoleon. Think and Grow Rich. 1. edition. Radford, VA: Wilder Publications, 2007 (originally published in 1937).

(82) Vujicic, Nick. Life without Limits: Inspiration for a Ridiculously Good Life. Colorado Springs, CO: Waterbrook Press, 2012.

CHAPTER TWELVE

GODDESS SELF-LOVE AND SELF-CARE

BEFRIENDING YOURSELF

What a martyr sees flash before her eyes before she dies: someone else's life. ~ Anon

I can think of no better way to end this book than with these two topics: self-love and self-care. We Goddesses do so much for the world, but we can't pour from an empty cup. We owe it to ourselves to nourish the most important relationship in our lives: the one we have with ourselves.

How are you treating yourself? Do you spend more time rewarding your wins or beating yourself up for your failures?

Self-Love

Self-love is appreciating YOU and valuing your own well-being and happiness. It's taking care of your own needs and not sacrificing your well-being to please others. Self-love means not settling for less than you deserve.

Self-love is individual and personal. What does it mean for you? It can mean:

- Holding yourself in high esteem.
- Keeping your inner dialogue positive.
- Putting yourself first.
- Trusting yourself to make good decisions.
- Forgiving yourself. Knowing that it's okay to make mistakes.
- Setting healthy boundaries.
- Not comparing yourself to others.
- Not worrying about others' opinions of you.
- Loving your body just as it is.
- Letting go of toxic people.
- Speaking your mind. Your thoughts matter. No less than the trees and the stars, you have a right to be here.
- Taking time to see the beauty around you.
- Going for your dreams.

Self-love means accepting who you are in this moment, the whole of your being.

Try This

Go to the nearest mirror, look yourself in the eyes, and say, "I love you. I really love you." Say it again with feeling. The harder that is to do, the more important it is to do it.

Create a vision board with images of things that you would like to bring into your life because they would bring you joy. Or buy a beautiful journal and use it to create a list that begins "I promise you, [your name] the following." Write a list of everything you want in life. A new wardrobe? A trip to Cancun? New socks? A calligraphy class? No matter how big or small it is, write it down and make a promise to yourself that these things will come, because you deserve them. Revisit this list every now and then. Add to it. Check off the items you've already achieved. You'll be surprised how often you do achieve them while forgetting you'd even committed them to the list!

And while you're making lists, create a list of all your accomplishments, everything you're proud of, and everything that's working for you in that moment. Add to this list over time.

We will never allow anyone to love us more than we love ourselves, so love yourself radically. When you wake up in the morning, give yourself a hug. Say, "I love you, [your name]." Do this any time you need a hug. Congratulate yourself when you complete a challenging task. Don't go on to the next task without recognizing your achievement and giving yourself encouragement. Say, "Great job, [your name]! You did it!"

We are too often our own worst critics. Let's instead be our greatest champions.

Self-Care

Self-care is self-love in action. It's anything you do for yourself to maintain your physical, mental, emotional, or spiritual health. Self-care benefits include increased resilience, better stress management, higher self-esteem, and a longer life. It also allows us to be kinder to others, and it shows others that we deserve to be treated well.

Anything that brings you sustained joy is self-care. It doesn't require that you spend money (though you certainly can).

Following are ways in which you can practice self-care.

- Spend more time in nature and less time online.
- Take yourself on play dates. In *The Artist's Way*, author Julia Cameron recommends two artist outings per week. Go to a museum, a textile mill, a glass blowing demonstration, the theater, a new bookstore, a nature walk, etc. Expand your horizons. You'll be amazed at the new interests you discover.
- Find something to be grateful for each day. Gratitude is the expression of love.
- Find a hobby you'd enjoy. Treat yourself to the classes, the tools, the time.
- Buy yourself fresh flowers (or cut them from your garden) and put them in the rooms you spend the most time in.
- Buy spa-quality bath towels and naturally scented bath salts.
- Make an appointment for a day of pampering at a day spa.

- Get a manicure or new hairstyle.
- Be intentional about what you put into or on your body. You deserve only the best, the freshest, the purest.
- Treat yourself to a dinner out. A friend of mine who had given up on finding true love decided to become her own true love. She got dolled up, made reservations at fine restaurants, and ordered whatever she wanted on the menu, including drinks with umbrellas in them. She eventually attracted the perfect mate, but that wasn't even her intention.
- Clear out your closet. When you purge outdated, worn, or unloved items you make room for those you love. If something has sentimental value but you know you'll never wear it, consider donating it with gratitude. As an article in MindBodyGreen.com stated, "Don't chase what's already happened; love yourself enough to know the best is yet to come."
- Go shopping for a new item to add to your wardrobe.
- Consider your spirituality. Even if you're not religious, believing in something beyond yourself helps build intuition and creates a sense of peace, love, and belongingness. Some non-secular books you might want to check out at your local library include *The Field* by Lynne McTaggart and *The Spontaneous Healing of Belief* by Gregg Braden. I also recommend *Proceed As Way Opens*, a compilation of seven years of spiritual blog entries by a lifelong student of philosophy, religion, meditation, and science. I helped to edit and publish this book as a ninetieth birthday gift to my spiritual mentor, friend, and author Reverend Billie Blain.
- Meditation is an enduring form of self-love. It is a gift you can give yourself any time as a break from stress, tension, and busyness. If someone you cared for was overexerting themselves, you'd recommend they take a break. Care for yourself enough to do the same.
- Exercise is another way to practice self-love. Taking care of your rarest possession—your own body—is crucial. Give yourself the gift of good health.

Stress Reduction

When stress overwhelms us, it can have toxic effects on our body. Therefore, stress reduction is a vital part of self-care. Stress reducing techniques may be short-term activities you can do anywhere, and include the following:

- **Guided imagery** is like taking a vacation in your mind. You can listen to an audio recording or create your own in your mind, imagining yourself walking through a peaceful scene that leads to a body of water or a clearing where you connect with Spirit, or merely spend time in solitude. I have a friend who calls this "going to my happy place" and used this when she had to have a breast biopsy, and later, chemotherapy treatments.
- **Meditation** provides both short-term stress relief and long-term stress management benefits.
- **Progressive muscle relaxation** is another way to reduce stress, particularly if the stress is causing tightness in your body. You practice this by tightening and then releasing each muscle group, starting with your head, and moving down to your toes. You should end with a feeling of relaxation throughout your body.
- **Listen to music:** Try going to YouTube and searching for a playlist of music from the year you graduated high school.
- **Ask for a hug** from a loved one or cuddle with your pet.
- **Try aromatherapy** through candles, diffusers, or other body products. Use natural products to avoid adding toxins to your environment.
- **Get an adult coloring book.** This saw a boost in popularity in the last few years for its stress-relieving benefits.

Longer-term activities include eating a balanced diet, ensuring you get regular leisure time, reining in your inner critic by reframing negative self-talk into positive self-talk, yoga, and gratitude.

Self-Care Areas

We are multifaceted beings! Self-care doesn't just mean taking a bubble bath, and it's not always just skin deep. Following are several areas where self-care might be needed, together with ideas for how you can express it.

- **Emotional self-care:** Journal, read uplifting books, listen to music, work out, take a walk, watch a comedy, cry, hug, or cuddle someone, take a nap.
- **Environmental self-care:** Take a walk, breathe in fresh air, enjoy the sun or night sky, pick up litter, recycle, clean your house, redesign a room.
- **Financial self-care:** Create a financial plan, open a savings account for a specific purpose (such as a trip), and cut back on unnecessary expenses that don't bring you joy.
- **Intellectual self-care:** Read, listen to audiobooks, watch documentaries, do crossword puzzles, try something new, take a class.
- **Occupational self-care:** Learn a new skill or trade, obtain a degree, polish your resume, apply for your dream job, open your own business. If you hate your job, care for yourself enough to find one you love.
- **Physical self-care:** Work out, get health check-ups, consider visiting a naturopath if you've never done so, floss and get your regular dental cleanings, reduce or eliminate alcohol, try to get 7-9 hours of sleep each night.
- **Social self-care:** Schedule regular outings with your friends. Reach out to friends you've lost touch with. Volunteer, get out, use social media wisely.
- **Spiritual self-care:** meditate, pray, reflect, take a yoga class, visit a holy site, be mindful, help those in need.

Self-care isn't something you do once and forget about. It should be a regular part of your day and your life. Treat yourself as the precious creature you are.

Goddess Gift: Homemade Bath Salts Recipe

- 4 cups Epsom salts
- 1 cup coarse dead sea salt or pink Himalayan salt crystals
- 40-60 drops of essential oils of your choice (see below)
- 4-6 tablespoons dried herbs or dried rose petals

Mix the above in a large bowl and store in an airtight glass container in the bathroom. Use a scoop to add 1-2 cups to your bath. For a sleep aid, use lavender and chamomile essential oils; for skin softening, use rose essential oil. For relaxation, use bergamot, neroli, and sandalwood essential oils. For rejuvenation, use eucalyptus, grapefruit, and clove.

THE PATH OF THE AGELESS GODDESS

The Goddess doesn't enter us from the outside; she emerges from deep within. ~ Marianne Williamson

The Ageless Goddess

- Aging is not a disease, merely a risk factor in age-related diseases.
- Chronological age and biological age are different. Biological age is almost entirely determined by lifestyle choices.
- Telomeres are structures at the ends of chromosomes that play a crucial role in cellular aging. Longer telomeres combat aging. Simple lifestyle changes can keep them long and strong.
- Inflammaging is chronic inflammation that can cause age-related disease. To prevent it, eat an anti-inflammatory diet, control blood sugar, maintain a healthy weight, and manage stress.
- Intermittent fasting can improve cellular health, lower insulin levels, fight inflammation, and reduce susceptibility to disease.
- While we can't change our genes, we can control which genes are expressed through lifestyle choices.

Goddess Nutrition

• A poor diet can cause high blood pressure, obesity, type 2 diabetes, high cholesterol and heart disease, stroke, gout, cancer, and
    premature death.
• The Mediterranean diet is one of the healthiest diets available.
• Aim for five servings of fruits and vegetables daily.
• Acidic cells lead to chronic pain, impaired metabolism, infections, and cancer.
• To determine your acidic/alkaline balance, purchase pH strips and measure both urine and saliva pH first thing in the morning. Aim for a tested pH of 6.5-7.3.
• Each produce color provides different nutritional benefits. Eat every color in the rainbow.
• Purchase organic food as much as possible, especially in coffee, wine, and the Dirty Dozen.
• Take a food-based multivitamin and consider taking a broad-spectrum probiotic for good gut health.
• Limit your consumption of large fish (tuna, swordfish) and avoid eating "farmed" fish, including farmed shrimp. Large fish contains higher levels of mercury; farmed fish contains contaminants. Eat only "wild-caught" fish.
• Most of us get too much omega-6 and not enough omega-3. Balance is crucial for health.
• Grass fed beef and butter and pasture-raised eggs are higher in omega-3 than are grain-fed.
• A well-balanced plate is half vegetables, one-quarter starch, and one-quarter protein.
• Include healthy fats (olive oil, coconut oil, eggs, avocado, nuts and seeds) when eating greens; they boost nutrient value.

Goddess Detox

* Remove fluoride, chlorine, and other contaminants from drinking and cooking water with a multi-step filtering system.
* Avoid plastic water bottles and don't use plastic/aluminum coffee pods.
* To avoid contact between plastic and food, first wrap food in parchment paper.
* Sweating is part of our body's natural detoxification system. Swap antiperspirant for deodorant.
* Radon is the #2 cause of lung disease, second only to smoking. Because radon is colorless and odorless, it's important to test the radon level of your home. Kits are available at most hardware stores.
* Ways to detox naturally include sweating, saunas, consuming cruciferous vegetables and probiotic foods, and intermittent fasting.
* Indoor plants help to purify the air in our homes. Aim for at least two good-size plants for every 100 square feet, and more is better!
* Glutathione is an antioxidant naturally produced by the body and it's crucial for detoxification. Foods that contain or boost glutathione include spinach, avocados, asparagus, okra, broccoli, Brussel sprouts, cauliflower, kale, watercress, mustard greens, shallots, and onions, Brazil nuts, poultry, beef, fish, cottage cheese, and organ meats. Turmeric and whey protein are contributors as well.

Goddesses Exercise

* Sitting for eight hours a day with no physical activity carries a risk of dying on par with that of smokers and obese individuals.
* One minute of exercise increases lifespan by a full seven minutes.
* Be sure you move your body every day for 30-60 minutes. This can be broken into several shorter sessions.
* Regular exercise keeps the hippocampus strong (the part of our brain responsible for memory).

- Rebounding is gentle on the joints. It boosts balance and coordination, supports pelvic floor health, and helps drain the lymphatic system.
- Strength training increases bone density and strengthens connective tissues, preventing fractures and other injuries. It decreases body fat, builds muscle mass, and improves mental health.
- For optimum health, include at least three vigorous aerobic workouts (or five moderate workouts), two strength workouts, and two balance and flexibility workouts each week.

Goddesses Hydrate

- Harvard Health researchers found that most people need at least four to six cups of water each day, not the eight cups we're usually told, and coffee and tea count. To be sure you're well hydrated, urine should be lemon-yellow.
- Carry water in a glass bottle, not plastic or aluminum.
- Avoid sports drinks, most of which are loaded with chemicals.

Goddess Healthcare

- All drugs have side effects, and drug interactions carry risk because it's difficult to calibrate medications appropriately when they're combined.
- Three medications that should be used with caution are acetaminophen (the active ingredient in Tylenol), linked to asthma and liver damage, steroids, which can destroy stem cells; and antibiotics, which can destroy gut flora.
- Medical screenings carry both risk and benefit and should be considered carefully in consultation with your medical provider.
- A UW-Madison study found that most women aged 50-74 should consider getting mammograms every three years instead of every two to reduce the risks associated with breast cancer screening.

Goddess Brain Power

- Dementia is not a normal part of aging. It is not something to fear, it is something to avoid.
- In only 1% of cases do genes determine whether a person will get Alzheimer's. These genes relate to amyloid-beta production. For the other 99% of cases, the causes are determined by lifestyle choices. And even for that 1%, the expression of genes is not fixed. Epigenetics is based on the understanding that we can modify the expression of our genes.
- Lifestyle choices to reduce one's chances of contracting Alzheimer's include not smoking, limiting alcohol consumption, eating a balanced diet with at least five servings of fruits and vegetables each day, limiting sugar, exercise, good sleep, and staying mentally and socially active.

Goddess Mindfulness and Mindset

- As the placebo effect demonstrates, we're not only what we eat, we're also what we think. Our inner dialogue, positive or negative, can impact our health at the cellular level.
- Benefits of positive self-talk include increases in vitality, satisfaction, immune function, physical wellbeing, and reductions in pain, stress, and risk of death.
- Mindfulness is awareness of the present moment, without judging. When we slow down and focus on the moment, we experience more joy and happiness in our lives.
- Meditation brings equanimity: mental calmness, composure, and evenness of temper, even in difficult situations.
- Meditation isn't the cessation of thinking; it's training yourself to remember to come back to the present (the breath or some other focal point).
- Meditation is as close as your own breath. Follow the breath from the inhale through the exhale and repeat. Even one minute a day (or several times a day) will reap many benefits.

- Health benefits of meditation include reducing blood pressure, helping our bodies recover from cortisol spikes (caused by stress) improving our immune function response, slowing age-related brain atrophy, and lessening the symptoms of depression and anxiety.
- Neuroscientists have found that meditation rewires the parts of the brain involved in self-awareness, compassion, and resiliency.

The Goddess in Nature

- We are evolutionarily wired to love natural settings and feel at peace there. Proximity to water has a naturally soothing effect.
- Spending more time in nature or at least outdoors (at least 150 minutes per week) can improve overall wellbeing. Time in nature helps reduce anxiety and depression.
- Finnish researchers found that merely sitting in nature made people feel psychologically restored, and when they walked in nature, the benefits were magnified.
- Even scenes and sounds of nature can have beneficial mental and physical effects.
- Adding houseplants to every room can help detoxify the air. The larger the leaf and soil exposure, the more purifying the plant.

Goddesses Connect

- Longevity experts now agree that the single biggest factor in living a long, healthy, and happy life is connectedness. Aim for four close friends, which can include your partner.
- Living with someone—even a non-intimate roommate—can decrease mortality risk by 10-32%. Volunteerism decreases it by 22%. Combining a happy marriage with connected friendships and a feeling of belongingness decreases mortality risk by 65%.
- One reason it's often hard to find new companions is that no one realizes that other people are looking, too! Loneliness is universal, but it's not incurable.

- *Kenzokin* is the Japanese term for people in our lives who are committed to our happiness and wellbeing. It means family, but not necessarily those who are blood relatives.
- *Ubuntu* is a South African word which means "I am because you are. My identity is such that it includes you. I would be a very different person without you."
- Friendship requires effort and time.
- To create closeness in a friendship, increase your understanding of the other (knowingness) and increase your investment in the other's well-being (caring).

Goddess Dreams and Goals

- Dreams and goals matter, and the second half of life is the perfect time to realize them.
- Personal development fosters better relationships, reduces stress, benefits our health, increases productivity, helps us self-regulate, breeds success, makes us more resilient, and increases feelings of contentment and happiness.
- For every excuse, there is a cure. Helen Keller said, "Life is either a daring adventure or nothing at all."

Goddess Self-Love and Self-Care

- We Goddesses do so much for the world, but we can't pour from an empty cup. We owe it to ourselves and others to nourish the most important
    relationship we have: the one we have with ourselves.
- Self-love is not selfish. It means taking care of your own needs and not sacrificing your well-being to please others.
- Self-love means accepting who you are in this moment, the whole of your being.
- Self-care is self-love in action. It's anything you do for yourself to maintain your physical, mental, emotional, or spiritual health.
- Stress reduction is a vital part of self-care. Ways to reduce stress and practice self-care include eating a balanced diet, honoring

leisure time, reining in your inner critic, and practice yoga and gratitude.

THANK YOU

Many thanks to *you*, my dear Goddess. Please spread the word to other Goddesses. Let's lift one another up in this life.

Thanks also to my review team of readers (you know who you are) and to my dear friend and author, Cate Read Hickman, my weekly writing companion. A big shout out to the Coterie of Hygge Queens. Everyone should have such a loving and creative group of friends and Goddesses!

And a big thanks to the staff at Beaverton City Library. I would be nowhere without your hold feature.

ABOUT THE AUTHOR

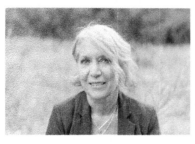 Yvonne Aileen is a nonfiction author and researcher. The goal of her Goddess series is to help women embrace their innate power in all areas of life. Her publishing house, 800 Muses (at 800Muses.com), raises women's voices through connection and cooperation. Ms. Aileen lives in Portland, Ore., with sons Max and Sam and canine writer's assistants Buddy and Daisy.

ALSO BY YVONNE AILEEN

AVAILABLE AS AUDIOBOOKS, EBOOKS, AND PAPERBACKS

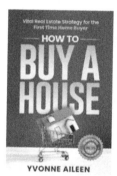 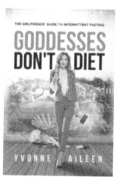 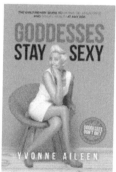

Releasing June 2022

For discounted bulk ordering in quantities of 10 or more, write publis her@800Muses.com.

Ms. Aileen is also a collaborating author for *Transforming Trauma: Inspiring Stories and Powerful Tools for Manifesting Peace, Hope, and Healing*. She has been a guest speaker on numerous podcasts and is available for speaking opportunities by writing publisher@800Muses. com.

A Favor, Dear Goddess

If you found value in this book, please take a moment to share your experience by leaving a review.

Made in the USA
Las Vegas, NV
03 February 2023

66807666R00095